Dermatology - Laboratory and Clinical Research

ACNE: CAUSES, TREATMENT AND MYTHS

DATE DUE

DERMATOLOGY - LABORATORY AND CLINICAL RESEARCH

Dermatology Research Focus on Acne, Melanoma and Psoriasis
David E. Roth (Editor)
2010. 978-1-60876-075-6

Acne: Causes, Treatment and Myths
Alexander K.C. Leung and K.I.E. Hon (Authors)
2010. 978-1-61668-258-3

Acne: Causes, Treatment and Myths
Alexander K.C. Leung and K.I.E. Hon (Authors)
2010. 978-1-61668-601-7

Dermatology - Laboratory and Clinical Research

ACNE: CAUSES, TREATMENT AND MYTHS

K.L.E. HON AND ALEXANDER K.C. LEUNG

Nova Science Publishers, Inc.
New York

LIBRARY OF CONGRESS CATALOGING-IN-PUBLICATION DATA

Available upon Request
ISBN: 978-1-61668-258-3

Published by Nova Science Publishers, Inc. New York

CONTENTS

PREFACE

Acne vulgaris is a highly prevalent, chronic inflammatory disease of pilosebaceous units. It is the most common skin disease affecting more than 85% of teenagers and young adults. It is not known how often these affected individuals would seek medical advice and treatment, but studies have shown that their quality of life can be severely compromised. The pathophysiology of acne involves increased production of sebum, proliferation of *Propionibacterium acnes* with resultant increase in chemotactic factors and pro-inflammatory mediators which lead to inflammation, release of lipids into the sebaceous duct and follicle, and obstruction of the pilosebaceous canal caused by hyperproliferation and shedding of keratinocytes in clumps. Hormonal and genetic factors also play major roles.

Acne can manifest in non-inflammatory or severe inflammatory forms. Acne tends to occur on but not limited to the face and the upper back. The pathognomonic lesion of acne is the comedo, which may be either open or closed. Inflammatory acne may take the form of erythematous papules, pustules, nodules, or cysts. The clinical course tends to be remitting. For most people, acne diminishes over time and tends to disappear after one reaches his or her early twenties.

Acne can be psychologically traumatic. Anxiety, depression and loss of social esteem have been reported. Depending on the severity of the acne, topical retinoids may be used alone or in combination with topical antibiotic and benzoyl peroxide. Oral antibiotics are an important therapy for the more inflammatory types of acne lesions, including papules, pustules, cysts, and abscesses. They should be used in combination with a topical retinoid or benzoyl peroxide. Oral isotretinoin should be reserved for resistant or scarring acne. The treatment should be adequately explained and compliance monitored. Specialist consultation is indicated in severe or unusual forms of acne such as acne conglobata, acne mendicamentosa and cosmetic acne.

INTRODUCTION

The term acne comes from the Greek word ἀκμή meaning a skin eruption. Acne refers to the presence of pustules and papules. The most common form of acne is known as "acne vulgaris", meaning "common acne". Many teenagers have this type of acne. Use of the term "acne vulgaris" implies the presence of comedones.

Acne vulgaris is a skin disease caused by changes in pilosebaceous units. A pilosebaceous unit is a skin structure consisting of a hair follicle and its associated sebaceous gland. Severe acne consists of an inflammatory component, but acne can also manifest in noninflammatory forms. Acne lesions are commonly referred to as pimples, blemishes, spots, zits, or acne. It is the most common skin condition during adolescence and affects more than 85% of teenagers, which often continues into adulthood [1]. Acne vulgaris is characterized by noninflammatory follicular papules or comedones and by inflammatory papules, pustules, and nodules in its more severe forms. Acne vulgaris affects areas of skin with the densest population of sebaceous follicles; these areas include the face, the upper part of the chest, and the back.

Acne is more common during adolescence presumably because of an increase in male sex hormones, which people of all genders accrue during puberty. For the majority of adolescents and young adults, acne diminishes over time and tends to disappear after one reaches his or her early twenties. There is, however, no way to predict how long it will take for acne to disappear entirely, and some individuals will continue to suffer well into their thirties and beyond.

Aside from scarring, main adverse effects are psychological, such as reduced self-esteem [2], depression, and suicidal tendency [3,4]. Acne usually appears during adolescence, when people already tend to be most socially insecure. The condition costs the community a substantial amount in resources [2]. It is a devastating disease striking most adolescents at their most vulnerable time when their life long self-esteem and sense of identity are being developed. Early and aggressive treatment is advocated by some authors to lessen the overall impact to individuals and society [2]. Currently available therapeutic agents are effective in suppressing inflammatory acne and preventing scarring in many patients. All clinicians caring for children and adolescents should be familiar with the pathogenesis, clinical manifestations, differential diagnosis, clinical evaluation, and treatment of acne. A review of the topic is therefore in order and is the purpose of the present publication.

It is noteworthy that some terms might be confused with acne. For instance, acne rosacea is a synonym for rosacea. Chloracne is associated with chlorine toxicity.

Chapter 1

EPIDEMIOLOGY

FREQUENCY AND RACIAL PREVALENCE

Acne vulgaris affects more than 85% of people at some time during their lives [1,5]. Acne tends to run in families. A family history of severe acne is associated with an earlier onset of acne, an increased number of retentional acne lesions and therapeutic difficulties [6].

The prevalence of acne in North Americans of African ancestry and whites is similar. Acne displays histological and clinical differences as well as response to therapeutic agents in people with different skin color [7]. Taylor and colleagues reported that papules were the most frequent presentation of acne in African Americans (70.7%) and Hispanics (74.5%); with Asians and other races having similar presentations [7]. Postinflammatory hyperpigmentation is often the chief complaint for acne in patients of darker races with acne.

Epidemiology of acne in other communities has also been studied. In the State of Victoria in Australia, the prevalence, severity and disability related to facial acne (comprising acne on the head and neck) were assessed in a randomized sample of 2491 students (aged 4 to 18 years) [8]. The overall prevalence (including 4 to 7 year olds) was 36.1% (95% confidence intervals [CI]: 24.7 to 47.5), ranging from 27.7% (95% CI: 20.6 to 34.8) in 10 to 12 year olds to 93.3% (95% CI: 89.6 to 96.9) in 16 to 18 year olds. It was less prevalent among boys aged 10 to 12 years than girls of the same age; however, between the ages of 16 and 18 years, boys were more likely than girls to have acne. Moderate to severe acne was present in 17% of students (24% boys, 11%

girls). Comedones, papules and pustules were the most common manifestations of acne, with one in four students aged 16 to 18 years having acne scars. Twelve per cent of students reported a high Acne Disability Index Score, which correlated with clinical severity, although there was some individual variation in perception of disability. Seventy per cent of those found to have acne on examination had indicated in the questionnaire that they had acne. Of those, 65% had sought treatment, a substantial proportion of affected individuals (varying with who gave the advice) was classified as being likely to have no beneficial effect. The study was the first population-based prevalence study on clinically confirmed acne published from Australia. The results show that acne is a common problem. The authors suggested the need for education programs in schools to ensure that adolescents understand their disease, and know what treatments are available and from whom they should seek advice.

There is some epidemiological evidence to suggest that incidence rates are considerably lower in non-westernized societies. Cordain et al reported the prevalence of acne in 2 non-westernized populations, the Kitavan Islanders of Papua New Guinea and the Ache hunter-gatherers of Paraguay, and analyzed how elements in non-westernized environments might influence the development of acne [9]. Of 1200 Kitavan subjects examined (including 300 aged 15 to 25 years), no case of acne (grade 1 with multiple comedones or grades 2 to 4) was observed. Of 115 Ache subjects examined (including 15 aged 15 to 25 years) over 843 days, no case of active acne (grades 1 to 4) was observed. The authors concluded that the astonishing difference in acne incidence rates between non-westernized and fully modernized societies cannot be solely attributed to genetic differences among populations but likely results from differing environmental factors. Identification of these factors may be useful in the treatment of acne in Western populations.

Prevalence and risk factors of facial acne vulgaris among Chinese adolescents have also been reported [10]. In the Guangdong Province, China, 3163 students 10 to 18 years old were selected from 7 schools. Information was collected using self-administrated questionnaires and physician examinations. The prevalence of acne vulgaris was calculated from the collected data. Potential risk factors including age, gender, diet, skin type, sleeping habits, and facial make-up use were analyzed using stepwise logistic regression. The results showed a prevalence of acne vulgaris of 53.5% in all adolescents, with 51.3% in males and 58.6% in females. The prevalence of inflammatory acne in males and females combined was 25.8% and of acne scarring 7.1%. Increased age was related to higher prevalence and severity of acne vulgaris: 15.6%, 44.9%, and 70.4% for 10, 13, and 16-year-olds, respectively. Acne vulgaris was more prevalent in girls under 14 years of age and boys over 14 years of age. Significant risk factors of acne vulgaris included age, skin type (oily, mixed, or neutral skin in comparison with dry skin), insufficient sleep, and cosmetic make-up use. The authors concluded that acne vulgaris is prevalent among Chinese 10 to 18 years.

The prevalence of facial acne in Peruvian adolescents and its relation to their ethnicity was described in a cross-sectional study of 2214 healthy adolescents (55.83% male and 44.17% female), 12 to 18 years old [11]. The adolescents studied were divided into three ethnic groups: whites, Mestizos, and Indians. Less than half of the adolescents (41.69%) had acne. The prevalence of acne in the adolescents of Arequipa was significantly less than that in Caucasians. Peruvian Indians had significantly less acne than Peruvian whites or Mestizos. The authors concluded that ethnicity is an important predictor of not only the prevalence, but also the severity of juvenile acne vulgaris in their sample.

AGE

The common forms of pediatric acne occur at two stages: in the newborn period and in adolescence. Acne vulgaris may be present in the first few weeks and months of life when a newborn is still under the influence of maternal hormones and when the androgen-producing portion of the adrenal gland is disproportionately large. Neonatal acne usually appears at 4 to 6 weeks of age and resolves spontaneously at 4 to 6 months of age. The lesions are in a distribution similar to that seen in adolescence, namely on the face, upper chest, and back. Infants with severe acne may develop severe acne during adolescence [12].

Adolescent acne usually begins prior to the onset of puberty, between ages 8 and 10 years in 40% of children, when the adrenal gland begins to produce and release more androgen hormone [13]. The early lesions are usually confined to the face and are primarily closed comedones. The prevalence of acne in boys increases from 40% at age 12 years to 95% at age 16 [14]. In girls, the prevalence increases similarly from 61% to 83% [14]. However, acne is not limited to adolescence. Twelve percent of women and 5% of men at age 25 years have acne. By age 45 years, 5% of both men and women still have acne.

Sex

Acne vulgaris is generally more common in males than in females during adolescence [8,11]. Acne tends to be more severe among males than females.

Chapter 2

PATHOGENESIS AND ETIOLOGY

The pathogenesis of acne vulgaris is multi-factorial. Four key factors are involved in the development of an acne lesion. These factors are follicular epidermal hyperproliferation with subsequent plugging of the follicle, excess sebum, presence and activity of *Propionibacterium acnes*, and inflammation.

Acne develops as a result of blockage in sebaceous follicles [1,13,15-18]. The stratum corneum lining of the follicles is overproduced due to androgen stimulation in adolescence. The presence of pilosebaceous ductal hypercornification can be seen histologically as microcomedones and clinically as blackheads, whiteheads, and other forms of comedones, such as macrocomedones. There is a significant correlation between the severity of acne and the number and size of microcomedones (follicular casts), the presence of which is a measure of comedogenesis [19]. The sebaceous follicles contain an enzyme 5α-reductase, which converts plasma testosterone to dihydrotestosterone. The latter is a potent stimulus for nuclear division of the follicular germinative cells and consequently of excessive cell production [15]. Thus, obstruction requires the presence of both circulating androgens and the converting enzyme.

Follicular epidermal hyperproliferation is the first recognized event in the development of acne. The exact underlying cause of this hyperproliferation is not known. Currently, several hypotheses have been proposed to explain why the follicular epithelium is hyperproliferative in individuals with acne. Firstly, androgen hormones have been implicated as the initial trigger. Comedones, the clinical lesion that results from follicular plugging, begin to appear around adrenarche in persons with acne. It has been shown that the degree of comedonal acne in prepubertal girls correlates with circulating levels of the adrenal androgen dehydroepiandrosterone sulfate (DHEA-S). Furthermore, androgen hormone receptors are present in the portion of the follicle where the comedone forms; individuals with malfunctioning androgen receptors do not develop acne.

Secondly, changes in lipid composition have been implicated in the development of acne vulgaris. Persons with acne frequently have excess sebum production and oily skin. This excess sebum may dilute the normal epidermal lipids and result in a change in the relative concentrations of the various lipids. Diminished concentrations of linoleic acid have been demonstrated in individuals with acne and, interestingly, these levels normalize after successful treatment with isotretinoin. This relative decrease in linoleic acid may be what initiates comedone formation [20].

Thirdly, inflammation is incriminated in comedone formation. Interleukin (IL)-1-α is a proinflammatory cytokine. It has been used in a tissue model to induce follicular epidermal hyperproliferation and comedone formation. Although inflammation is not apparent microscopically or clinically in early lesions of acne, it may still play a pivotal role in the development of acne vulgaris and the comedones.

Fourthly, excess sebum is a key factor in the development of acne vulgaris. Sebum production and 'excretion are regulated by a number of different hormones and mediators. Androgen hormones, in particular, promote sebum production and release. Yet most men and women with acne have normal circulating levels of androgen hormones. An end-organ hyperresponsiveness to androgen hormones has been hypothesized. Numerous other agents, including growth hormone and insulin-like growth factor, also regulate the sebaceous gland and may contribute to the development of acne.

The pathogenesis of inflammatory acne is less well understood [1,13,16-18,21-23]. Inflammation may be a primary phenomenon or a secondary phenomenon. Most of the evidence to date suggests a secondary inflammatory response to *P. acnes* (vide supra). However, IL-1-α expression has been identified in the microcomedone, and it may play a role in the development of acne. Physical manipulation of a closed comedo could certainly lead to rupture of the cavity contents into the dermis, with a subsequent inflammatory response. Spontaneous inflammation also occurs in obstructed follicles, but the reason for this is unclear. An attractive hypothesis is that over-growth of gram-positive bacteria in the obstructed follicle (either *P. acnes* or *Staphylococcus epidermidis*) might stimulate factors that initiate inflammation [21]. In the study by Leyden et al, Propionibacterium species were quantified on the foreheads and cheeks of persons with and without acne in three age groups: 11

to 15, 16 to 20, and 21 to 25 years of age. Propionibacteria were virtually absent in the pubertal non-acne group compared to a geometric mean density of 114,800 per sq cm in the acne group. A similar sharp difference existed between the acne subjects and normal subjects in the age range of 16 to 20 years: 85,800 organisms per sq cm compared to 588 per sq cm. Patients with acne and normal subjects over age 21 showed no difference in Propionibacterium levels [21].

P. acnes is a microaerophilic organism present in many acne lesions. Although *P. acnes* has not been shown to be present in the earliest lesions of acne, its presence in later lesions is almost certain. *P. acnes* stimulates inflammation by producing proinflammatory mediators that diffuse through the wall of the hair follicle. Recent studies have shown that *P. acnes* activates the toll-like receptor 2 on monocytes and neutrophils [24]. Activation of the toll-like receptor 2 then leads to the production of multiple proinflammatory cytokines, including IL-12, IL-8, and tumor necrosis factor. Hypersensitivity to *P. acnes* may also explain why some individuals develop inflammatory acne vulgaris while others do not. Superantigen from *P. acnes* triggers inflammation of comedones in genetically predisposed individuals [1,13,16-18,25-33]. Further evidence of the role that *P. acne* plays in the pathophysiology is evident in photoinactivation of *P. acnes* by near-ultraviolet light [34] and in eradication of *P. acnes* by its endogenic porphyrins after illumination with high intensity blue light [35]. *P. acnes*-induced mediators of inflammation are inhibited by many Indian herbs [36]. Overproduction of sebum and free fatty acid formation seem unlikely as causes of inflammation in acne.

Other mechanisms may also be involved in the pathophysiology in adolescence. Acne may result from several external causes. Fictional acne may be caused by headbands, football helmets, or tight-fitting brassieres or other garments. Oil-based cosmetics may be responsible for predominantly comedonal acne, and hair sprays may produce acne along the hair margin.

Drugs responsible for acne include glucocorticoids, androgens, hydantoins, lithium, iodides, and isoniazid, possibly mediated by increased plasma testosterone. Drug-induced acne should be suspected in teenagers if all lesions are in the same stage at the same time and if involvement extends to the lower abdomen, lower back, arms, and legs. Some cosmetic agents and hair pomades have been reported to exacerbate acne.

Hyperkeratinization and formation of a plug of keratin and sebum (a microcomedo) is the earliest change. Enlargement of sebaceous glands and an increase in sebum production occur with increased androgen (DHEA-S) production at adrenarche. The microcomedo may enlarge to form an open comedo (blackhead) or closed comedo (whitehead). Whiteheads are the direct result of skin pores becoming clogged with sebum and dead skin cells. In these conditions the naturally occurring commensal bacteria *P. acnes* can cause inflammation, leading to inflammatory lesions (papules, infected pustules, or nodules) in the dermis around the microcomedo or comedo.

A number of morphologically different inflammatory lesions may form that can be painful and unsightly. In 30% of patients, such lesions lead to scarring [37]. Reactive oxygen species generated by neutrophils may have a role in mediating acne inflammation. Metronidazole, which is effective in the treatment of acne, markedly inhibits reactive oxygen species generated by neutrophils. The drug is known to have no significant effect on the growth of *P. acnes*. The proportion of linoleic acid is markedly decreased in acne comedones. Linoleic acid significantly suppresses reactive oxygen species generated by neutrophils. The ability of neutrophils to produce reactive oxygen species is significantly increased in patients with acne inflammation [38]. In the study by Akamatsu et al, patients with acne inflammation showed a significantly increased level of hydrogen peroxide produced by neutrophils compared to patients with acne comedones and healthy controls [39]. There were no marked differences in the level of hydrogen peroxide produced by neutrophils between patients with acne comedones and healthy controls. In addition, patients with acne inflammation treated by oral administration of minocycline hydrochloride showed a significant decrease in the ability of neutrophils to produce hydrogen peroxide with resultant decrease in the inflammatory activity of acne lesions. The study suggested that acne inflammation is mediated in part by hydrogen peroxide generated by neutrophils.

There is ample clinical evidence suggesting that emotional stress can influence the course of acne [40,41]. Substance P and other neuropeptides may stimulate lipogenesis of the sebaceous glands which may be followed by proliferation of *P. acnes*, and may yield a potent influence on the sebaceous glands by provocation of inflammatory reactions via mast cells. Thus, cutaneous neurogenic factors should contribute to the onset and/or exacerbation of acne inflammation.

Role of hormones in pilosebaceous unit development has been described [42]. Androgens such as testosterone, dihydrotestosterone and DHEAS are important in the pathogenesis of acne. Medical disorders such as congenital adrenal hyperplasia, polycystic ovary syndrome, and other endocrine disorders with excess androgens may trigger the development of acne vulgaris.

Although androgens are required for sexual hair and sebaceous gland development, pilosebaceous unit growth and differentiation require the interaction of androgen with numerous other biological factors. Hair follicle growth involves close reciprocal epithelial-stromal interactions that recapitulate ontogeny; these interactions are necessary for optimal hair growth in culture. Peroxisome proliferator-activated receptors and retinoids have recently been found to specifically affect sebaceous cell growth and differentiation. Many other hormones such as growth hormone, insulin-like growth factors, insulin, glucocorticoids, estrogen, and thyroid hormone play important roles in pilosebaceous unit growth and development [43]. Menopause-associated acne occurs as production of the natural anti-acne ovarian hormone estradiol fails at menopause. Improved understanding of the multiplicity of factors involved in normal pilosebaceous unit growth and differentiation may aid in the provision of optimal treatment for these patients.

Acne may result from sebaceous gland dysfunction. A strong increase in sebum excretion occurs a few hours after birth; this peaks during the first week and slowly subsides thereafter. A new rise takes place at about age 9 years with adrenarche and continues up to age 17 years, when the adult level is reached. The sebaceous gland is an important formation site of active androgens. Androgens are well known for their effects on sebum excretion, whereas terminal sebocyte differentiation is assisted by peroxisome proliferator-activated receptor ligands. Estrogens, glucocorticoids, and prolactin also influence sebaceous gland function. In addition, stress-sensing cutaneous signals lead to the production and release of corticotrophin-releasing hormone from dermal nerves and sebocytes with subsequent dose-dependent regulation of sebaceous nonpolar lipids. Other sebaceous gland dysfunctions are also associated with the development of acne, including sebaceous proinflammatory lipids; different cytokines produced locally; periglandular peptides and neuropeptides, such as corticotrophin-releasing hormone, which is produced by sebocytes; and substance P, which is expressed in the nerve endings at the vicinity of healthy-looking glands of acne patients [41].

Chapter 3

MYTHS AND MISUNDERSTANDING

Many factors such as smoking, pre-menstruation, stress, sleep deprivation, cosmetics, excessive sweating and drugs (such as steroids, diphenylphenytoin, phenobarbital, isoniazid, etc) have been implicated as aggravating factors, and sunshine or ultraviolet light as protective factors [44,45].

The prevalence and demographic factors of acne in a general population sample and the association of smoking and acne on a qualitative and quantitative level has been investigated [44]. In a cross-sectional study, 896 citizens of the City of Hamburg were dermatologically examined. The prevalence and severity of acne were recorded and further information on demographic variables, medical history, and alcohol and cigarette consumption were obtained by a standardized interview. According to the clinical examination, acne was present in 26.8% overall, and was more prevalent in men (29.9%) than women (23.7%) (odds ratio [OR]: 1.37; 95% CI: 1.01 to 1.87). Prevalence followed a significant linear trend over age with peak prevalence between 14 and 29 years ($p < 0.001$). The reported age at onset was significantly lower in women than men ($p = 0.015$). According to multiple logistic regression analyses acne prevalence was significantly higher in active smokers (40.8%, OR: 2.04; 95% CI: 1.40 to 2.99) as compared with non-smokers (25.2%). A significant linear relationship between acne prevalence and number of cigarettes smoked daily was obtained (trend test: $p < 0.0001$). A significant dose-dependent relationship between acne severity and daily cigarette consumption was shown by linear regression analysis ($p = 0.001$). The authors concluded that smoking is a clinically important contributory factor to acne prevalence and severity

Although acne is a common dermatological disorder with an underlying hormonal basis, studies to determine the ways in which the different stages of the menstrual cycle affect acne in women are rare. In one study, 400 females, aged 12 to 52 years, were questioned whether their acne got worse before, during, or after their menstrual period and they were also asked whether the acne was related to the menstrual period [45]. Their age, severity of acne, ethnicity, and oral contraceptive use were also recorded. One hundred seventy seven of 400 (44%) of those interviewed experienced premenstrual flares of their acne. Severity of acne, ethnicity, and oral contraceptive use did not affect the premenstrual flare rate. Women older than 33 years had a higher rate of premenstrual flares relative to women aged 20 to 33 years (p = 0.03 by chi^2 analysis). The authors concluded that almost half of all women experience premenstrual flares of their acne. Premenstrual flares may be more common in older women [45].

Food has also been implicated and many patients hold the belief that their acne is influenced by dietary factors, while in previous decades, doctors thought that diet had little influence on acne [46-50]. There is surprisingly little good scientific evidence to support or refute the role of diet in the pathogenesis of acne [47,51]. One of the foods that has received a lot of medical attention is milk. Recently, three epidemiological studies from the same group of scientists found an association between acne and consumption of partially skimmed milk, instant breakfast drink, sherbet, cottage cheese, and cream cheese [51-53]. The researchers hypothesized that the association may be caused by hormones (such as several sex hormones and bovine IGF-1) or even iodine present in cow milk [20]. They reasoned that some of these products survive digestion and could have biological effects in humans.

Adebamowo et al examined data from the Nurses Health Study II to retrospectively evaluate whether intakes of dairy foods during high school were associated with physician-diagnosed severe teenage acne [51]. The investigators studied 47,355 women who completed questionnaires on high school diet in 1998 and physician-diagnosed severe teenage acne in 1989, and estimated the prevalence ratios and 95% confidence intervals of acne history across categories of intakes. After accounting for age, age at menarche, body mass index, and energy intake, the multivariate prevalence ratio (95% CI; P value for test of trend) of acne, comparing extreme categories of intake, were: 1.22 (1.03 to 1.44; 0.002) for total milk; 1.12 (1.00 to 1.25; 0.56) for whole milk; 1.16 (1.01 to 1.34; 0.25) for low-fat milk; and 1.44 (1.21 to 1.72; 0.003) for skim milk. Instant breakfast drink, sherbet, cottage cheese, and cream cheese were also positively associated with acne. The authors found a positive association with acne for intake of total milk and skim milk, and hypothesized that the association with milk may be because of the presence of hormones and bioactive molecules in the milk

In a subsequent prospective cohort study, Adebamowo and colleagues evaluated 6,094 girls, aged 9 to 15 years, who reported dietary intake on up to three food frequency questionnaires from 1996 to 1998 [52]. Presence and severity of acne were assessed by questionnaires in 1999. The authors computed multivariate prevalence ratios and 95% confidence intervals for acne. After accounting for age at baseline, height and energy intake, the multivariate prevalence ratios (95 % CI; p-value for test of trend) for acne comparing highest (2 or more servings per day) to lowest (<1 per week) intake categories, were 1.20 (1.09 to 1.31; <0.001) for total milk, 1.19 (1.06 to 1.32; <0.001) for whole milk, 1.17 (1.04 to 1.31; 0.002) for low fat milk and 1.19 (1.08 to 1.31; <0.001) for skim milk, respectively. The results did not change appreciably when girls who reported use of contraceptives were excluded and analysis was restricted to those younger than 11 years of age at baseline. The authors found a positive association between intake of milk and acne. This finding supports their earlier studies and suggests that the metabolic effects of milk are sufficient to elicit biological responses in consumers [52]. The authors further sought to examine the association between dietary dairy intake and acne among male teenagers in a prospective cohort study. They studied 4273 boys, members of a prospective cohort study of youths and of lifestyle factors, who reported dietary intake on up to 3 food frequency questionnaires from 1996 to 1998 and teenaged acne in 1999 [53]. They computed multivariate prevalence ratios and 95% confidence intervals for acne. After adjusting for age at baseline, height, and energy intake, the multivariate prevalence ratios (95% CI; P value for test of trend) for acne comparing highest (>2 servings/d) with lowest (<1/wk) intake categories in 1996 were 1.16 (1.01 to 1.34; 0.77) for total milk, 1.10 (0.94 to 1.28; 0.83) for whole/2% milk, 1.17 (0.99 to 1.39; 0.08) for low-fat (1%) milk, and 1.19 (1.01 to 1.40; 0.02) for skim milk. Acne assessment was by self-report and boys whose symptoms might have been part of an underlying disorder were not excluded. The authors did not adjust for steroid use and other lifestyle factors that might affect occurrence of acne. The authors found a positive association between intake of skim milk and acne. This finding suggests that skim milk contains hormonal constituents, or factors that influence endogenous hormones, in sufficient quantities to have biological effects in consumers [53].

Apart from protein food sources, carbohydrates have also been implicated. The long-held belief that there is no link between diets high in refined sugars and processed foods and acne has recently been challenged [47]. The previous belief was based on earlier studies (based on the consumption of chocolate and Coca Cola) that were methodologically flawed [42,47,54]. Acne is caused by the action of dihydrotestosterone, derived from endogenous and exogenous precursors, likely acting synergistically with IGF-1 [55]. The more recent low glycemic-load hypothesis postulates that rapidly digested carbohydrate foods (such as soft drinks, sweets, white bread) produce an overload in blood glucose (hyperglycemia) that stimulates the secretion of insulin, which in turn triggers the release of IGF-1 [47]. IGF-1 has direct effects on the pilosebaceous unit and has been shown to stimulate hyperkeratosis and epidermal hyperplasia [56]. These events facilitate acne formation. Sugar consumption might also influence the activity of androgens via a decrease in sex hormone-binding globulin concentration [57,58]. In support of this hypothesis, a randomized controlled trial showed that a low glycemic-load diet improved acne and reduced weight, androgen activity and levels of insulin-like growth factor binding protein-1 [59]. High IGF-1 levels and mild insulin resistance (which causes higher levels of insulin) have been observed in patients with acne [9,60,61]. High levels of insulin and acne are also both features of polycystic ovarian syndrome [47]. According to this hypothesis, the absence of acne in some non-Westernized societies could be explained by the low glycemic index of these cultures' diets [11]. It is possible that genetic reasons account for the rarity of acne in these populations, although similar populations (such as South American Indians or Pacific Islanders) do develop acne [9,62]. Further research is necessary to establish whether a reduced consumption of high-glycemic foods, or treatment that results in increased insulin sensitivity (like metformin) can significantly alleviate acne [56,57,63,64].

Observational evidence suggests that dietary glycemic load may be one environmental factor contributing to the variation in acne prevalence worldwide. To investigate the effect of a low glycemic load (LGL) diet on endocrine aspects of acne vulgaris, Smith et al conducted a parallel, controlled feeding trial involving a 7-day admission to a housing facility on 12 male acne suffers (17.0 ± 0.4 years) [56]. Subjects consumed either a LGL diet (n = 7; 25% energy from protein and 45% from carbohydrates) or a high glycemic load (HGL) diet (n = 5; 15% energy from protein, 55% energy from carbohydrate). Study outcomes included changes in the homeostasis model assessment of insulin resistance (HOMA-IR), sex hormone binding globulin (SHBG), free androgen index (FAI), IGF-I, and its binding proteins (IGFBP-I and IGFBP-3). Changes in HOMA-IR were significantly different between groups at day 7 (-0.57 for LGL vs. 0.14 for HGL, p = 0.03). SHBG levels decreased significantly from baseline in the HGL group (p = 0.03), while IGFBP-I and IGFBP-3 significantly increased (p = 0.03 and 0.03, respectively) in the LGL group. These results suggest that increases in dietary glycemic load may augment the biological activity of sex hormones and IGF-I, and that these diets may aggravate potential factors involved in acne development

In a recent study, Smith et al determined the effect of a low glycemic load diet on acne and the fatty acid composition of skin surface triglycerides [64]. Thirty-one male acne patients (aged 15 to 25 years) completed sebum sampling tests as part of a 12-week, parallel design dietary intervention trial. The experimental treatment was a low glycemic load diet, comprised of 25% energy from protein and 45% from low glycemic index carbohydrates. In contrast, the control group received carbohydrate-dense foods without reference to the glycemic index. Acne lesion counts were assessed during monthly visits. At baseline and 12-weeks, the follicular sebum outflow and composition of skin surface triglycerides were assessed using lipid absorbent tapes. At 12 weeks, subjects on the experimental diet demonstrated increases in the ratio of saturated to monounsaturated fatty acids of skin surface triglycerides when compared to controls [5.3 ± 2.0% (mean ± S.E.M.) vs. -2.7 ± 1.7%, P = 0.007]. The increase in the saturated/monounsaturated ratio correlated with acne lesion counts (r = -0.39, P = 0.03). Increased follicular sebum outflow was also associated with an increase in the proportion of monounsaturated fatty acids in sebum (r = 0.49, P = 0.006). Their study suggests a possible role of desaturase enzymes in sebaceous lipogenesis and the clinical manifestation of acne. The lesson from the aforementioned studies suggested that consumption of high-glycemic foods should be kept to a minimum and avoidance of "junk food" with its high fat and sugar content.

Smith and colleagues compared the effect of an experimental low glycemic-load diet with a conventional high glycemic-load diet on clinical and endocrine aspects of acne vulgaris [57]. A total of 43 male patients with acne completed a 12-week, parallel, dietary intervention study with investigator-masked dermatology assessments. Primary outcomes measures were changes in lesion counts, sex hormone binding globulin, free androgen index, IGF-1, and insulin-like growth factor binding proteins. At 12 weeks, total lesion counts had decreased more in the experimental group (-21.9 [95% CI: -26.8 to -19.0]) compared with the control group (-13.8 [-19.1 to -8.5], P = 0.01). The experimental diet also reduced weight (P = 0.001), reduced the free androgen index (P = .04), and increased insulin-like growth factor binding protein-1 (P = 0.001) when compared with a high glycemic-load diet. The limitation of this study was that the investigators could not preclude the role of weight loss in the overall treatment effect. The finding suggests nutrition-related lifestyle factors play a role in acne pathogenesis.

Along the dietary dimension, vitamin deficiencies have also been implicated. Low plasma levels of vitamin A and E have an important role in the pathogenesis of acne and in the aggravation of this condition. Studies have shown that newly diagnosed acne patients tend to have lower levels of vitamin A circulating in their bloodstream than those who are acne free [65]. In addition people with severe acne also tend to have lower blood levels of vitamin E [65].

Lay perceptions that diet, hygiene and sunlight exposure are strongly associated with acne causation and exacerbation are common but at variance with the consensus of current dermatological opinion. Magin et al reviewed the literature to assess the evidence for diet, face-washing and sunlight exposure in acne management [66]. Original studies were identified by searches of the Medline, EMBASE, AMED (Allied and Complementary Medicine), CINAHL, Cochrane, and DARE databases. Methodological information was extracted from identified articles but, given the paucity of high quality studies found, no studies were excluded from the review on methodological grounds. Given the 'prevalence of lay perceptions, and the confidence of dermatological opinion in rebutting these perceptions as myths and misconceptions, surprisingly little evidence exists for the efficacy or lack of efficacy of dietary factors, face-washing and sunlight exposure in the management of acne. Many of the studies have methodological limitations. Based on the existing evidence, the investigators remarked that clinicians cannot be didactic in their recommendations regarding diet, hygiene and face-washing, and sunlight to patients with acne. Advice should be individualized, and both clinician and patient cognizant of its limitations.

Wuthrich et al studied 120 patients with acne vulgaris using an intracutaneous allergen test with 23 of the most important food allergens [67]. The skin test results of 83 patients (69.2%) were negative, only 9 (7.4%) showed a distinct immediate reaction on four or more food extracts. Almonds showed the most positive reactions (11.6%), followed by malt (10%), cheese (8.3%), mustard (8.3%), red pepper (8.3%), and wheaten flour (7.5%). Thereupon the patients were instructed to either keep no diet at all, or to follow an acne diet, or a special elimination diet based on the results of the skin testing. In addition, all the patients had to undergo the same mild acne local therapy. After 3 months of treatment (with monthly controls) only 45 patients could be evaluated. No statistical difference was found within the three groups with regard to the success of treatment. Diet prescriptions for acne vulgaris are generally not very significant, although they are possibly useful in individual cases.

Many young people with acne hold beliefs that they have problems with personal hygiene. It is important to realize that acne is definitely not caused by dirt or due to poor personal hygiene. This misconception probably comes from the fact that blackheads look like dirt stuck in the openings of pores. As aforementioned under the section of pathophysiology, the black color is not dirt but simply oxidized keratin. In fact, the blockages of keratin that cause acne occur deep within the narrow follicle channel, where it is impossible to wash them away. These plugs are formed by the failure of the cells lining the duct to separate and flow to the surface in the sebum. Built-up oil of the skin can block the passages of these pores, so standard washing of the face could wash off the oil and help unblock the pores.

CLINCIAL MANIFESTATIONS

There are almost as many classifications of acne as there are clinicians with particular interest in the disease. Thus acne has been classified as types I-IV, inflammatory versus noninflammatory, comedonal, comedopapular, papular, papulopustular, pustular, and "cystic" or nodular (even nodular-cystic). For those who are enamored of classification, there are subdivisions of the various categories, including "sandpaper comedones" and microcysts. There is even disagreement as to what constitutes a papule versus a nodule. The classic textbook definition of a nodule refers to lesions 1 cm or larger, but the early investigators of oral isotretinoin defined nodules as 4 mm or larger, and this definition has incorporated into many textbooks [68].

Acne lesions tend to occur on the face, and to a less extent, on the upper back, chest, and shoulders. These areas correspond to the distribution of the largest and most numerous pilosebaceous units in the body [19,68,69]. The distal extremities are always spared.

The pathognomonic lesion of acne is the comedo, which may be either open or closed. An open comedo, also called a blackhead, is a flat or slightly raised black lesion, measuring 1 to 3 mm in diameter. The black surface of the open comedo is melanin, not dirt or oxidized fat. The pigmentation is limited to the tip of the comedo because melanocytes are present only in the upper portion of the sebaceous follicle. A closed comedo, commonly known as a whitehead, appears as a pale, slightly elevated papule without a readily visible central pore. It is flask-shaped with the narrowest portion connected to the skin surface.

Blackheads do not generally become inflamed unless the pilosebaceous canal is disrupted by external forces, such as may occur by squeezing the lesion [19,68,69]. Whiteheads may either open up their pores resulting in blackheads or they may evolve into papules and pustules. For this reason, closed comedones have been called "the time bombs of acne". With rupture of the obstructed follicle and release of free fatty acids into the surrounding tissue, an inflammatory reaction ensues, resulting in erythematous papules, pustules, nodules, or cysts depending on the amount and location of the tissue involved, and the magnitude of the inflammatory response. Mild inflammatory acne is characterized by inflammatory papules and comedones. On the other hand, moderate inflammatory acne is characterized by comedones, inflammatory papules, and pustules.

Nodulocystic acne is characterized by comedones, inflammatory lesions and large nodules greater than 5 mm in diameter. Acne conglobata is a severe, destructive and highly inflammatory form of acne marked by the presence of multiporous comedones, nodules, cysts, abscesses, and draining sinus tracts on the upper trunk and posterior back [70]. The condition is rare in children and it predominantly affects adult males. Acne conglobata may develop into acne inverse in adulthood, which is chronic, severe and non self-healing. Multiple draining sinuses are often present in intertriginous areas, leading to hypertrophic scars and skin contractures. The lesions are highly resistant to treatment and excision may be necessary.

Acne fulminans is a rare form of acne characterized by the sudden eruption of large, necrotic, ulcerating nodulocystic lesions on the back and chest in association with systemic manifestations such as fever, chill, malaise, weight loss, musculoskeletal pain, polyarthralgia, leukocytosis, anemia, elevated erythrocyte sedimentation rate, and osteolytic bone lesions [71,72]. Lytic lesions in the bones of the anterior chest wall and in the epiphyseal growth plates are common in patients with acne fulminans, but do not seem to occur in patients with severe cystic acne. The prognosis of bone disease associated with acne fulminans appears to be good, and the chronic sequelae, if any, are mild sclerosis and hyperostosis of the affected bones. Acne fulminans should be added to the list of dermatoses associated with bone lesions detectable by radiologic and scintigraphic methods [72].

Although acne is a disease in adolescent, there are a few subtypes typified by age (vide infra) [69]. Neonatal acne is more common in boys than girls and onset can be as early as the first few days or weeks of life. Individual lesions are similar to adolescent acne but mainly on the face and seldom on the trunk. The condition may be associated with sebaceous hyperplasia of nose and cheeks. Neonatal acne may occur with fetal hydantoin syndrome [73].

Chapter 4

DIFFERENTIAL DIAGNOSIS

The differential diagnosis of acne varies by age and, in some cases, may warrant a work-up in order to rule out underlying systemic abnormalities. In atypical cases of acne vulgaris, angiofibromas, flat warts, and acne rosacea need to be considered [74].

Angiofibromas (adenoma sebaceum) are composed of vascular and connective tissue elements and are found in approximately 75% of patients with tuberous sclerosis. The lesions typically appear during preschool years in the malar area as small pink or red dome-shaped papules in a "butterfly distribution". The lesions gradually enlarge and become more numerous with age.

Flat warts (verruca plana) are small, slightly elevated flat-topped papules with a finely roughened surface. They may be differentiated from closed comedones which have a dome shape and a smooth surface. Flat warts vary in size whereas closed comedones are uniformly small.

Acne rosacea is an acneiform eruption affecting the face in middle-aged and older persons. It can be distinguished from acne by the presence of telangiectasia and the absence of comedones.

In neonatal acne, differential diagnosis includes candidiasis, nevus comedonicus, and steroid acne. Neonatal acne almost always resolves spontaneous before 3 months of age [75]. Adrenal hyperplasia should be considered if the condition persists beyond one year of age, especially in girls.

In infantile acne, there is a male predominance and onset is at 3 to 12 months of age [75,76]. Differential diagnosis includes candidiasis, nevus comedonicus, and steroid acne, and the patient should be evaluated for 21-OH hydroxylase deficiency if the acne is severe [77]. Mid-childhood acne is very rare. Onset is at 3 to 8 years. Hyper-androgenism needs to be ruled out.

Women who present with acne in conjunction with hirsutism, alopecia or menstrual disturbances should be examined for the possibility of ovarian or adrenal hyperandrogenism [78,79].

Chapter 5

CLINICAL EVALUATION

The history should include the time of onset, duration, severity, as well as the types and distribution of acne lesions. One should also evaluate the degree of local as well as systemic symptoms [19,68,69,80]. Local symptoms may include pain or tenderness. Systemic symptoms are most often absent except in acne fulminans. The use of previous acne medications, including over-the-counter preparations and their effect, should also be noted. A history of the use of cosmetics, moisturizers, body lotions, shampoos, and hair pomades may be helpful in defining exacerbating factors. The history of past health and present medical illness including menstrual disorders should be obtained. The impact of acne on the patient's quality of life should be explored [81].

The physical examination should include an assessment of the number, type, and distribution of the lesions [19,68,69]. Because acne lesions may vary in number during the natural course of the disease, various measurements have been developed based on clinical examination and photographic documentation. These measurements range from global assessments to counting of lesions; the latter provide more objective data [82].

Many systems for grading the severity of acne have been used. Generally, the severity of acne is assessed by the number, type, and distribution of lesions [82]. The Leeds acne grading technique, counts and categorizes lesions into inflammatory and non-inflammatory (ranges from 0 to 10.0) [83]. The Cook's acne grading scale uses photographs to grade severity from 0 to 8 (0 being the least severe and 8 being the most severe). The Pillsbury scale simply classifies the severity of the acne from 1 (least severe) to 4 (most severe). In a study evaluating Allen and Smith grading scale, two 12-week-long double-blind placebo-controlled studies of acne treatments were performed using three judges and a total of 331 male college students [84]. Global severity grades and papule, pustule, and comedo counts were performed every two weeks. The data were evaluated using Pearson's coefficient of correlation, and results showed a high degree of correlation between global severity grades and lesion counts, as well as among judges. These data suggest that acne grading scales and papule counts are equally reproducible methods of grading inflammatory acne and that the comedo grading scale and comedo count are equally reproducible methods of grading comedonal acne [84]. The Pillsbury scale simply classifies the severity of the acne from 1 (least severe) to 4 (most severe) [82].

The growth parameters and sexual development should also be noted. Special attention should be paid to signs of androgen excess such as hirsutism, polycystic ovaries, and obesity.

Chapter 6

ASSESSMENT OF PSYCHOSOCIAL IMPACT

Psychological assessment is important. Acne is perceived by adolescents to have important negative personal and social consequences, and that improvement in these areas may follow medical treatment [81]. The Acne-Specific Quality of Life Questionnaire (Acne-QoL) is a useful tool in the assessment of the psychosocial impact on the patient's quality of life.

In order to measure the impact of facial acne across four dimensions of patient quality of life, Acne-QoL was utilized in two randomized, double-blind, placebo-controlled studies of the efficacy of Estrostep (norethindrone acetate/ethinyl estradiol) in the treatment of facial acne [85]. A total of 296 Estrostep and 295 placebo patients were evaluated. The Acne-QoL was completed at the beginning, middle (cycle 3), and end (cycle 6) of the 6-month treatment period. The responsiveness of the Acne-QoL was demonstrated through its ability to detect both small (baseline to mid-study) and moderate (baseline to study end) treatment advantages for Estrostep patients. Confirmatory factor analysis supported the subscale structure, and internal consistency estimates were excellent. Convergent and discriminant validity were supported by correlations between Acne-QoL scores and clinical measures that were both in the direction and relative magnitude hypothesized. Finally, item response theory analyses confirmed that each item is highly related to its subscale's latent construct and that each subscale is sensitive across a broad range of the underlying continuum. The study results confirm that the Acne-QoL is responsive, internally consistent, and valid [85]. Screening tools for depression in acne vulgaris patients are also available [86].

Chapter 7

LABORATORY INVESTIGATIONS

Routine laboratory testing is not necessary. If there is evidence of hyperandrogenism (e.g. irregular menses, androgenic alopecia, or hirsutism), serum DHEA-S and free testosterone levels should be measured [87]. If these levels are elevated, an evaluation of adrenal and gonadal function is indicated. An elevated serum free testosterone level indicates a hyperandrogenous state of adrenal or ovarian origin; an increased DHEA-S level suggests adrenal hyperandrogenism and an LH/FSH ratio of greater than 3 suggests polycystic ovary syndrome. Investigations are usually not necessary in typical cases unless severe acne occurs in atypical sites, the age of onset is between 1 and 6 years, or there are signs of hyperandrogenism (Cushingoid features, cliteromegaly, precocious puberty, hirsutism, increased libido, deepening of voice). If these signs are present, the patient should be screened for congenital adrenal hyperplasia, polycystic ovarian syndrome, iatrogenic cause (athletes taking hormones) and genetic diseases (such as XYY syndrome) [87].

Chapter 8

COMPLICATIONS

Post-inflammatory erythema and pigmentation may result and may last for several months. Scarring may also result, especially with the severe variants such as acne conglobata and acne fulminans. In general, the deeper the inflammatory process, the more likely it will result in permanent scarring. Scarring can vary from small, deep punched-out pits ('ice-pick' scars) to deep furrows, keloid, and hypertrophic scars [88].

Acne can also lead physical pain and discomfort. A severe inflammatory variant of acne, acne fulminans, can be associated with fever, arthritis, and other systemic symptoms.

Acne can lead to psychosocial disturbance (vide supra) [3,81]. Acne occurs at a time of life when personal appearance is very important and self-consciousness is at its peak. Self-consciousness related to acne can have an adverse effect on dating, participation in social activities, and quality of life. Acne may also be associated with suboptimal employment and financial prospects [89]. In some individuals, the psychological scars can be greater than the physical scars. A New Zealand study showed that young people presenting with acne were at increased risk of depression, anxiety and suicide attempts. 'Problem acne' was associated with an increased probability of depressive symptoms, odds ratio 2.04 (95% CI: 1.70 to 2.45); anxiety, odds ratio 2.3 (95% CI: 1.74 to 3.00); and suicide attempts, odds ratio 1.83 (95% CI: 1.51 to 2.22) in a logistic model that included age, gender, ethnicity, school decile and socio-economic status. The association of acne with suicide attempts remained after controlling for depressive symptoms and anxiety, odds ratio 1.50 (95% CI: 1.21 to 1.86) [3]. Suicidal ideation was reported in 7.1% of acne patients [4]. As acne is more common in women than in men during adulthood, the authors concluded that the psychosocial impacts may be more pronounced in the females. In another study, Picardi et al estimated the prevalence of suicidal ideation among patients with dermatologic conditions, and to identify demographic, clinical, and psychosocial correlates [4]. Two samples of outpatients with dermatologic conditions (n = 294) and inpatients (n = 172) completed the 12-item General Health Questionnaire, the Skindex-29, and the Patient Health Questionnaire. Forty patients (8.6%) reported suicidal ideation during the previous 2 weeks. In univariate analysis, the presence of suicidal ideation was associated with female sex, inpatient status, presence of a depressive or anxiety disorder, and higher 12-item General Health Questionnaire and Skindex-29 scores. The size of the diagnostic groups allowed reasonable prevalence estimates only for psoriasis (10%) and acne (7.1%). In multivariate analysis, only emotional distress (12-item General Health Questionnaire) and impaired social functioning (Skindex-29) were independently associated with suicidal ideation. The authors admitted that they lacked an observer-rated evaluation of skin condition and could rely only on the Skindex-29 symptoms subscale as a measure of disease severity. In addition, the measurement of suicidal ideation was limited as a result of the use of only one question to assess it. Furthermore, the cross-sectional design prevented causal inferences. The authors concluded that suicidal ideation is not rare among patients with dermatologic conditions. Assessing suicidality would be warranted in dermatologic practice among patients at particular risk such as women with high psychologic distress and impaired social functioning. The development of psychiatric consultation-liaison services is mandatory to provide effective treatment and careful follow-up of patients who have suicidal tendency [4].

Chapter 9

PREVENTION

Under normal circumstances, dietary factors play only a minor role in the pathogenesis of acne. It is a common misconception that certain foods, particularly chocolate, pizza, fried food, fatty foods, and nuts make acne worse. Studies have failed to show a relationship with these dietary facts. Notwithstanding this evidence, if an individual relates an exacerbation of acne to certain foods, a trial of avoidance is appropriate.

Since acne is not caused by uncleanliness, frequent washing of the face will not prevent or clear acne. Obsessive scrubbing with soap may actually worsen the condition. Nevertheless, the face should be washed whenever it is oily and approximately twice a day otherwise. Mild soaps are preferred.

Many cosmetics are capable of inciting acneiform changes. Make-up should be avoided. If cosmetics are used, water-based products instead of occlusive, oil-based products are preferred and they should be used sparingly.

Pinching or popping acne lesions may rupture the pilosebaceous canal and produce larger and more persistent lesions. These practices should be discouraged.

MANAGEMENT

Numerous publications have been written on the subject matter of management of acne. The mechanisms of acne formation and the treatment plans must be explained to the patients [117]. Treatment regimens must be individualized depending on severity and presence of inflammatory acne or scarring [5,19,24,68,69,74,80,90-121]. The goals of treatment are to provide the patient with the best appearance possible and to minimize scarring [122-124]. The aims of therapy are to prevent follicular hyperkeratosis, reduce *P. acnes*, inhibit sebum secretion and fatty acid production, and eliminate comedones.

Time spent at the first visit to answer questions is important. It is important to explain that there will not be much improvement for 4 to 8 weeks, and no drug will prevent an adolescent from ever having another acne lesion. A written education sheet is useful.

There are many products available for the treatment of acne, but many of which are without any scientifically-proven effects. Treatment regimens should be simple [125]. Complex regimens are expensive and associated with problems of skin irritation and compliance. Treatments are believed to work in at least 4 different ways (with many of the treatments providing multiple simultaneous effects) including normalizing of follicular epidermal hyperproliferation, killing *P. acnes*, anti-inflammatory effects, and hormonal manipulation. A combination of treatments can greatly reduce the amount and severity of acne in many cases. Those treatments that are most effective tend to have greater potential for side effects and the need for a greater degree of monitoring. Hence, a step-wise approach is preferred. Patients should consult with their doctors when deciding which treatments to use, especially when considering using treatments in combination. The mainstay of acne therapy is the use of potent topical keratolytic agents applied to the skin to relieve follicular obstruction. Depending on the severity of the acne, topical retinoids may be used alone or in combination of another agent such as topical antibiotic and benzoyl peroxide. This regimen will control 80 to 85% of cases of adolescent acne. Systemic treatment is necessary to prevent significant psychological and social impairment in these patients. Significant inflammatory and nodulocystic acne is usually recalcitrant to topical treatment, whereas uncommon acne variants, such as acne fulminans, pyoderma faciale, and acne conglobata, need to be promptly and effectively controlled. In all of these circumstances, systemic agents are indispensable. The choices include oral antibiotics, isotretinoin, and hormonal treatment [118,126].

Follow-up visits are essential. The criterion for ideal control is a few lesions every 4 weeks. During the visits, it may be necessary to explain again what medications are being used and what the treatment is intended to achieve. Patients should be questioned to determine whether the medications are being used properly.

Topical Keratolytics and Bactericidals

Topical treatment is usually the first line of treatment for acne [127]. Benzoyl peroxide is one of the most commonly prescribed topical agents used in mild to moderate acne. The medication should be applied to both affected and unaffected skin so as to treat missed comedones and microcomedones [128]. Care must be taken when using benzoyl peroxide, as it can very easily bleach any fabric or hair it comes in contact with. It may be used either alone or in combination with topical or systemic antibiotics and/or retinoids. The gel or cream containing benzoyl peroxide is rubbed, twice daily, into the pores over the affected region. Bar soaps or washes may also be used and vary from 2 to 10% in strength. Benzoyl peroxide is converted to benzoic acid and oxygen in the skin. The antibacterial effect on *P. acnes* is due to the oxidation of bacterial proteins. Benzoyl peroxide inhibits the lipolysis of sebum triglycerides and decreases the inflammation of acne lesions [129]. In addition, it has a comedolytic effect [129]. Unlike antibiotics, benzoyl peroxide has the advantage of being a strong oxidizer and thus does not appear to generate bacterial resistance. The major reported side effects are localized dryness, erythema, and peeling which, in most patients, will disappear with continued use. A sensible regimen may include the daily use of low-concentration (2.5%) benzoyl peroxide preparations for short contact (30 min) on alternate days, combined with suitable non-comedogenic moisturizers to help avoid over drying the skin. The concentrate can be increased and changed to daily treatment. However, dose-response studies are lacking. Various strengths of aqueous gel, lotion, cream, and wash are available. Efficacy is generally comparable to topical antibiotics [130,131].

Topical azelaic acid is mainly antibacterial but also has mild keratolytic effects [108,132]. It is suitable for mild, comedonal acne. It may cause initial stinging but additional whitening effect may be beneficial for post-inflammatory hyperpigmentation. Topical azelaic acid cream helps both to normalize keratinization and to reduce the proliferation of *P. acnes*, and has proven to be effective against both noninflammatory and inflammatory lesions. The results of a recent study have shown that its efficacy can be enhanced, and patient ratings of overall impression improved, when it is used in combination with other topical medications such as benzoyl peroxide 4% gel, clindamycin 1% gel, tretinoin 0.025% cream, and erythromycin 3%/benzoyl peroxide 5% gel [125,132]. Azelaic acid plus benzoyl peroxide achieves greater efficacy and higher patient ratings of convenience than monotherapy with erythromycin-benzoyl peroxide gel [132].

Topical Antibiotics

Topical antibiotics are used to avoid the side effects caused by systemic antibiotics, such as upset stomach and drug interactions [133]. Topical antibiotics that have been used successfully in the treatment of acne include erythromycin, clindamycin, stievamycin, and tetracycline. One percent clindamycin phosphate solution is the most efficacious topical antibiotic [133]. Topical erythromycin cream or lotions (1.5% and 4%) is also effective and clinical improvement is usually noted within 2 weeks but use up to 3 months is necessary to achieve maximum effect [133]. The major drawback in the use of topical antibiotics is the emergence in bacterial resistance. The risk of pseudomembranous colitis from the absorption of topical clindamycin is low. Topical tetracycline has been reported to stain the skin yellow. In addition, a bizarre fluorescence under fluorescent light has also been reported with topical tetracycline.

Topical antibiotics should not be used as monotherapy, because combination with topical retinoids or benzoyl peroxide will provide better results and will reduce antibiotic resistance [130]. Clindamycin/benzoyl peroxide gel has demonstrated efficacy and good overall tolerability in several well designed clinical studies in the topical treatment of patients with mild to moderately severe acne vulgaris [134]. In a randomized, double-blind comparison of a clindamycin phosphate/benzoyl peroxide gel formulation and a matching clindamycin gel with respect to microbiologic activity and clinical efficacy in the topical treatment of acne vulgaris, the total *P. acnes* count (P = 0.002) and the clindamycin-resistant *P. acnes* count (P = 0.018) were significantly reduced after 16 weeks of treatment with the combination gel compared with clindamycin monotherapy. These reductions in total *P. acnes* and clindamycin-resistant *P. acnes* counts correlated with reductions in total acne lesions [135]. A new combination formulation that contains 1% clindamycin and 5% benzoyl peroxide (BenzaClin Topical Gel) is available. In clinical trials, clinical improvement occurred at the first two follow-up visits and continued throughout treatment [136]. In addition, combination therapy with clindamycin/benzoyl peroxide gel rapidly reduces *P. acnes* counts and suppresses the emergence of clindamycin-resistant *P. acnes*. This formulation is stable at room temperature for up to 2 months after compounding. The aqueous gel vehicle is less drying, and there is no photosensitivity associated with its use. Clindamycin/benzoyl peroxide gel is an effective topical agent in the treatment of patients with mild to moderately severe acne, especially if the acne is caused by resistant strains of *P. acnes*. It is a suitable alternative for patients who are currently using topical antibacterials either alone or in conjunction with other topical anti-acne agents or systemic antibacterials [134].

Topical erythromycin with and without zinc is clinically effective, and both preparations produce significant reductions in acne grade, and inflamed and non-inflamed lesion counts [137]. Topical erythromycin is less effective than oral antibiotics [138], but efficacy is similar to topical clindamycin [139]. Combination of erythromycin with benzyl peroxide has good bactericidal effect [140,141], and combination with tretinoin is also available. In a double-blind clinical study in 94 subjects, a 1.5% (w/v) erythromycin lotion was as effective as 5% (w/v) benzoyl peroxide gel in significantly reducing the number of small inflamed lesions and the overall acne severity. However, benzoyl peroxide also significantly reduced the number of non-inflamed lesions whereas erythromycin had no effect on such lesions [131]. Topical antibiotics offer the advantages of decreased total absorption and, therefore, a corresponding decrease in systemic side effects compared with systemic antibiotics. Like systemic antibiotics, topical antibiotics act by decreasing colonization with *P. acnes* and by inhibiting neutrophil chemotaxis. Patients should be advised that improvement may take several months to develop. Side effects include dryness and local irritation from the vehicle in which the antibiotics are contained. Resistant staphylococci and *P. acnes* become more common during therapy but decrease after treatment stops [142,143].

Systemic Antibiotics

Oral antibiotics are an important therapy for the more inflammatory types of acne lesions, including pustules, cysts, and abscesses [118,129,144-146]. They should be used in combination with a topical retinoid or benzoyl peroxide. Tetracyclines are the first line antibiotics and macrolides are the second line. These antibiotics, administered systemically, produce a significant reduction in *P. acnes*. These antibiotics are concentrated in the sebum and are therefore very effective in inflammatory acne. In addition, they have intrinsic anti-inflammatory properties, exerting their action through the inhibition of neutrophil chemotaxis and alteration of macrophage and cytokine production [129,144].

The usual dosage of tetracycline and minocycline is 0.5 to 1 g and 50 to 100 mg, respectively, taken one hour before or two hours after meal. Tetracycline is contraindicated in pregnancy and it may cause staining of teeth in children under the age of twelve years. The most common side effects of tetracycline are mild gastrointestinal upsets and monilial vaginitis. Because tetracycline may cause esophageal ulceration when swallowed dry, the medication should be taken with a large glass of water. Other side effects include drug eruptions, photosensitivity, hepatotoxicity, onycholysis, pseudotumor cerebri, and gram-negative folliculitis [147]. Liver function should therefore be monitored during treatment. It is important to note that tetracycline should not be given with vitamin A or oral isotretinoin. The combined use is associated with increased risk of benign intracranial hypertension. Tetracycline can interact with anticonvulsants, anticoagulants, digoxin, lithium and theophylline, and may reduce efficacy of oral contraceptive pills [148].

Minocycline is a semi-synthetic tetracycline analogue [149]. It should be avoided in patients with a personal or family history of systemic lupus erythematosus. The usual dosage is 100 to 200 mg daily. Absorption is less affected by food than oxytetracycline. Side effects include vertigo, tinnitus, lupus erythematosus-like syndrome with polyarthritis. Minocycline may cause reversible blue-black pigmentation [150]. The pigmentation commonly first noted on shins. It may be localized on acne, scars, mucous membranes, teeth, nails [151], or generalized [152]. It is not the first line drug due to reported cases of lethal hypersensitivity reactions [153,154]. Pseudotumor cerebri can be induced by minocycline therapy [155]. Doxycycline is the second most active tetracycline analogue. The usual dosage is 100 mg daily. Its efficacy is equal to minocycline but with more antibiotic resistance. It is less binding to calcium and causes less dental changes [156]. Oral absorption is unaffected by food.

The macrolides represent second line oral antibiotics for acne. Erythromycin is a preferred option if patients might become pregnant or is breast-feeding or for children less than 8 years of age when tetracyclines are contraindicated. The usual dosage is 0.5 to 1 g per day in two divided doses for 6 months. The most common side effects of erythromycin are gastrointestinal upsets such as nausea, vomiting, abdominal cramps, diarrhea, and moniliasis. Oral erythromycin therapy can be followed by 1 to 2 months of topical antibiotic as maintenance [153,154,157-161].

Azithromycin enjoys good compliance due to few side effects. It is taken 250 mg once a day, 3 times per week [162]. Singhi et al conducted a non-randomized controlled trial on 70 outpatients with acne vulgaris to compare the efficacy and safety of azithromycin and doxycycline in the treatment of inflammatory acne [163]. In the first group, azithromycin was administered 500 mg daily before meals for 3 consecutive days in a 10-day cycle, with the remaining seven days in each cycle being drug-free days. The second group was given doxycycline 100 mg daily after meals. Topical erythromycin was prescribed to all patients. Clinical assessment was done at 10-day intervals for both the groups up to three months. They followed the severity index described by Michaelsson for assessment of outcome measures. There was 77.26% improvement in azithromycin treated group in comparison to 63.74% in the doxycycline treated group. There was a statistically significant reduction in severity in the azithromycin treated group. The study showed that a combination of azithromycin with topical erythromycin was significantly better than doxycycline with topical erythromycin in the treatment of acne vulgaris. The incidence and severity of side effects were also lower with azithromycin

Trimethoprim has also been used in dosage of 400 to 600 mg/day in two divided doses but has fallen out of favor because bacterial resistance is common [164].

A 6-month course of oral antibiotic is usually prescribed in association with topical therapy. Repeated course, preferably with the same antibiotic to reduce antibiotic resistance, may be required. Another antibiotic may be tried if no response is apparent in 3 months. Combinations of antibiotic usage include gastrointestinal.upset and development of resistance which is common with erythromycin and rare with minocycline [146].

Hormonal Treatments

Hormonal therapy is an important component in the treatment of women with acne who may or may not have elevated serum androgens [43,87,165]. The mainstays of hormonal therapy include oral contraceptives and antiandrogens such as cyproterone acetate, flutamide or spironolactone. Lucky et al compared the efficacy of a low-dose combined oral contraceptive (COC) containing 3-mg drospirenone and 20-microg ethinyl estradiol (3-mg DRSP/20-microg EE) administered in a 24-day active pill/4-day inert pill (24/4) regimen and placebo in women with moderate acne vulgaris during 6 treatment cycles [166]. A total of 534 participants were randomized and dispensed study medication (n = 266 [3-mg DRSP/20-microg EE 24/4 regimen COC group]; n = 268 [placebo group]). Women of reproductive age were eligible for inclusion in the study. Treatment with the 3-mg DRSP/20-microg EE 24/4 regimen COC was associated with a greater reduction from baseline to end point in individual lesion counts (papules, pustules, open and closed comedones) compared with placebo. The mean nodule count remained essentially constant throughout the study and was low in both treatment groups. There was a significantly higher probability that a participant had an improved assessment on the investigator's overall improvement rating scale (OR: 4.02; 95% CI: 2.29 to 7.31; P < .0001) and participant's overall self-assessment rating scale (OR: 2.82; 95% CI: 1.60 to 5.13; P = .0005) in the 3-mg DRSP/20-microg EE 24/4 regimen COC group than in the placebo group. The authors concluded that COC 3-mg DRSP/20-microg EE 24/4 regimen is a suitable option for women with moderate acne vulgaris who require contraception.

Although hormones are important in the development of acne, many questions remain unanswered regarding the mechanisms by which hormones exert their effects. It is not known whether these hormones are taken up from the serum by the sebaceous gland, whether they are produced locally within the gland, or whether a combination of these processes is involved. Finally, the cellular and molecular mechanisms by which these hormones exert their influence on the sebaceous gland have not been fully elucidated. Hormonal therapy is an option in women with acne not responding to conventional treatment or with signs of endocrine abnormalities [42,43,87,165].

Topical Retinoids

Topical retinoids are mainstay of acne treatment [167-171]. Depending on the severity of the acne, topical retinoids may be used alone or in combination of another agent such as topical or oral antibiotic and benzoyl peroxide. Topical retinoids are comedolytic; they normalize desquamation of keratinocytes by affecting follicular epithelial turnover and cell maturation. They also have intrinsic anti-inflammatory properties; they inhibit migration of inflammatory cells and release of inflammatory mediators. Topical retinoids improve the penetration of other topical agents and may minimize residual hyperpigmentation in dark skin individuals after resolution of inflammatory lesions. For best results, topical retinoids should be initiated at the onset of therapy. They should be applied at least 15 minutes after washing and on thoroughly dry skin. As with other topical medications used for the treatment of acne, topical retinoids should be applied as a thin layer to all acne-prone areas rather than to individual lesions. The sensitive periorbital and perioral areas, however, should be avoided. Patients should be advised that improvement may be delayed for 2 to 3 months after starting therapy. The major side effects are dryness, erythema, burning sensation, and irritation. In general, alcohol-based gels are more irritating than cream-based products. Topical retinoids also cause thinning of the stratum corneum which may predispose to sunburn and accelerate the carcinogenic effect of sunlight [1]. Sunscreens are necessary in patients who are unable to avoid exposure to sun. Topical retinoids often cause an initial flare up of acne and facial flushing. This can be prevented by starting from low concentration and increasing strength monthly as necessary, withholding drug for a few days and apply mild topical steroid. Topical retinoids are contraindicated in pregnancy and contraceptive precautions are needed in child-bearing age group [172].

Retinoids include tretinoin (brand name Retin-A), adapalene (brand name Differin), and tazarotene (brand name Tazorac). First generation topical retinoids are all-trans retinoic acid. Tretinoin (Retin A®) is an example which comes in 0.025%, 0.05%, 0.1% cream and 0.01%, 0.025% gel. Skin irritation may occur and treatment may be temporarily stopped. Isotretinoin (Isotrex®) is an example of second generation topical retinoid. It is a 13-cis retinoic acid. That is less irritating than tretinoin but the action is the same as first generation topical retinoic acid. Adapalene (Differin®) is an example of the third generation top which is a naphthoic acid derivative with retinoid receptor binding activity [173]. It possesses anti-inflammatory effect and is less irritating than tretinoin. Topical application of isotretinoin and adapalene has proved effective in treating acne vulgaris. Both drugs demonstrate therapeutic advantages and less irritancy over tretinoin, the most widely used treatment for acne. They both act as retinoid agonists, but differ in their affinity profile for nuclear and cytosolic retinoic acid receptors. In a randomized open-label clinical trial comparing topical adapalene gel 0.1% vs. isotretinoin gel 0.05% in the treatment of acne vulgaris, the two gels studied demonstrated comparable efficacy. Significantly lower skin irritation was noted with adapalene, indicating that adapalene may begin a new era of treatment with low-irritant retinoids [174].

Tazarotene gel is an effective, safe, and generally well-tolerated therapy for the treatment of acne vulgaris [175]. A randomized vehicle-controlled trial of short-contact therapy with 0.1% tazarotene gel demonstrated that tazarotene gel therapy is a safe and effective new method of acne treatment [176]. Furthermore, the efficacy and tolerability of tazarotene 0.1% gel and tretinoin 0.1% microsponge gel were evaluated in a multicenter, double-blind, randomized, parallel-group study in patients with mild-to-moderate inflammatory facial acne vulgaris [177]. One hundred sixty nine patients were randomized to once-daily applications of one of these topical retinoids for 12 weeks. Both agents were associated with significant reductions from baseline in the noninflammatory and inflammatory lesion counts. Tazarotene treatment was associated with a significantly greater incidence of treatment success (defined as $\geq$ 50% global improvement [67% vs 49%; P = 0.03]) and significantly greater reductions in overall disease severity (36% vs 26%; P = 0.02) and noninflammatory lesion count (60% vs 38% at week 12; P = 0.02) than tretinoin microsponge treatment. Both drugs were well tolerated, with mean levels of dryness, burning, pruritus, erythema, and peeling generally being no more than trace throughout the study. There were no clinically significant between-group differences in these measures of tolerability. Two patients in each group (2%) discontinued because of treatment-related adverse events. The mean amount of medication applied by the patients was 0.28 g per application with tazarotene and 0.41 g per application with tretinoin microsponge, resulting in cost-effectiveness ratios of $81.45 per treatment success with tazarotene and $108.24 per treatment success with tretinoin microsponge. Tazarotene was observed to have greater efficacy and comparable tolerability and to be a cost-effective alternative to tretinoin 0.1% microsponge gel.

Many comparative studies have also been performed. In a multicenter, double-blind, randomized comparison study of the efficacy and tolerability of once-daily tazarotene 0.1% gel and adapalene 0.1% gel for the treatment of facial acne vulgaris, tazarotene 0.1% gel was more effective than adapalene 0.1% gel and was also a more cost-effective treatment option [125].

In a noninferiority study of adapalene 0.1% gel versus tazarotene 0.1% cream in treating acne, 202 subjects 12 to 35 years of age with acne vulgaris participated in a 12-week, randomized, evaluator-blinded study of once-daily therapy with adapalene 0.1% gel versus tazarotene 0.1% cream [178]. The primary measure of efficacy was the reduction in total lesion counts posttreatment. Subjects treated with adapalene 0.1% gel achieved similar reductions in total lesion counts at week 12 compared to the subjects treated with the tazarotene cream, which demonstrates the noninferiority of adapalene treatment compared to tazarotene (median difference: -1.18%; lower confidence limit [LCL]: -9.26). At week 2, the number of patients that experienced erythema and scaling with tazarotene 0.1% cream was greater when compared to adapalene 0.1% gel and statistically significant. By week 12, the percentage of subjects reporting cutaneous irritation had returned to or near baseline levels and was similar between treatment arms for all parameters assessed. Adapalene gel was associated with fewer treatment-related adverse events than tazarotene cream (36% versus 58%, respectively), and less than half as many adverse events that were "definitely" related to study treatment than tazarotene cream (20% versus 45%, respectively). Daily therapy with adapalene 0.1% gel was shown to be noninferior to tazarotene 0.1% cream in total acne lesion reductions, and during initial stages of treatment, demonstrated better tolerability with respect to erythema and scaling

Thiboutot et al evaluated the efficacy and tolerability of a new, higher concentration of adapalene, adapalene 0.3% gel, compared to tazarotene 0.1% gel in the treatment of acne vulgaris [179]. The primary efficacy outcome was the percent reduction in total lesion count at week 12. Subjects 12 to 35 years of age with acne vulgaris (n = 172) participated in a 12-week, randomized, evaluator-blinded, noninferiority study of once-daily therapy with adapalene 0.3% gel or tazarotene 0.1% gel. Subjects in each group achieved clinically significant reductions in total lesion counts at week 12 (61% and 57% median reductions for adapalene and tazarotene, respectively); adapalene 0.3% gel was noninferior to tazarotene 0.1% gel (95% CI: -5.2 to -9.6). The adapalene arm was also therapeutically similar to the tazarotene arm in terms of the percent reduction in inflammatory and noninflammatory lesion counts at week 12, as well as in the assessments of acne severity and improvement. Mean tolerability scores for erythema, dryness, scaling, and stinging/burning were consistently lower in the adapalene arm compared to patients treated with tazarotene ($P < 0.014$ at week 12, Cochran-Mantel-Haenszel [CMH] test). The worst score for any tolerability parameter in the treatment phase in the adapalene arm was less than 1 (mild). Adapalene was also associated with a lower incidence of treatment-related adverse events when compared to tazarotene (3.5% versus 14%, respectively). Once daily therapy with adapalene 0.3% gel provided similar efficacy (non-inferior) to tazarotene 0.1% gel in the treatment of acne vulgaris, but demonstrated a superior tolerability profile.

Double strength Isotrexin (isotretinoin 0.1% w/w and erythromycin 4.0% w/w) versus Benzamycin (benzoyl peroxide 5.0% w/w and erythromycin 3.0% w/w) in the topical treatment of mild to moderate acne vulgaris was also evaluated [180]. The treatments were comparable with regard to their effects on inflammatory and non-inflammatory lesions and acne grade. Few adverse events were considered to be treatment-related. Both the isotretinoin/erythromycin and benzoyl peroxide/erythromycin gels were generally well tolerated. Compliance was better with the isotretinoin/erythromycin gel, which had the advantages of not requiring mixing or storage in a refrigerator, and was applied once rather than twice daily. The investigators concluded that isotretinoin/erythromycin gel given only once daily showed comparable efficacy with benzoyl peroxide/erythromycin given twice daily in the treatment of mild to moderate acne vulgaris of the face.

Optimizing the use of tazarotene for the treatment of facial acne vulgaris through combination therapy has been further studied [181]. Draelos et al performed a multicenter, investigator-masked, randomized, parallel-group study in 440 patients with mild-to-moderate facial acne vulgaris to compare the efficacy and tolerability of tazarotene monotherapy with 3 combination regimens - tazarotene plus benzoyl peroxide gel, tazarotene plus erythromycin/benzoyl peroxide gel, and tazarotene plus clindamycin phosphate lotion [181]. An additional treatment group, monotherapy with clindamycin phosphate lotion, also was included as a reference arm. The only combination therapy to achieve a significantly greater global improvement than tazarotene monotherapy was tazarotene plus clindamycin. For reducing noninflammatory lesions specifically, none of the combination regimens offered significant benefit over tazarotene monotherapy (though tazarotene plus clindamycin and tazarotene plus erythromycin/benzoyl peroxide were significantly more efficacious than clindamycin monotherapy). For reducing inflammatory lesions, tazarotene plus erythromycin/benzoyl peroxide was significantly more efficacious than all the other regimens. Although tazarotene plus clindamycin and tazarotene plus benzoyl peroxide reduced the incidence of adverse effects compared with tazarotene monotherapy, the difference did not achieve statistical significance.

Some dermatologists initiate adapalene gel treatment first, due to its good tolerability, followed by a switch to tazarotene cream in an effort to improve or hasten efficacy outcomes. A study by Gold et al compared the efficacy and safety of 2 daily regimens for the treatment of acne: adapalene 0.1% gel for 12 weeks and adapalene 0.1% gel for 6 weeks followed by tazarotene 0.1% cream for 6 weeks [182]. The primary efficacy outcome was the percent of reduction in total lesion counts post-treatment. Subjects ages 12 to 35 years with acne vulgaris were selected to participate in a 12-week, randomized, evaluator-blind study of once-daily therapy with adapalene 0.1% gel (n = 101) or "switch therapy," adapalene 0.1% gel followed by tazarotene 0.1% cream (n = 100). Adapalene-treated subjects achieved similar percent reductions in total lesion counts at week 12 compared to subjects receiving switch therapy, demonstrating the noninferiority of adapalene gel treatment (median difference: -3.57%; lower confidence limit [LCL]: -11.25). Adapalene gel was associated with fewer reports of cutaneous irritation, particularly for scaling and stinging/burning, and fewer treatment-related adverse events compared to switch therapy. The results of this study indicated that daily therapy with adapalene 0.1% gel for 12 weeks was non-inferior to switch therapy. Nowadays, "switch therapy" is no longer considered necessary and most physicians would simply use adapalene alone.

Oral Retinoids

The oral retinoid, 13-cis- retinoic acid (isotretinoin; Accutane), is the most effective treatment for severe cystic acne. Peck et al randomized 33 patients with treatment-resistant cystic and conglobate acne in a double-blind fashion to test the efficacy of isotretinoin versus placebo [70]. There was an overall 57% increase in the number of cystic lesions in 17 patients who initially received placebo. Sixteen of these 17 patients then received isotretinoin, with a resultant 98% improvement. The 16 patients who had been randomly assigned to receive initial therapy with isotretinoin had a 95% improvement. Twenty-seven of the 32 patients treated with isotretinoin had their acne cleared completely. The average maximum dosage of isotretinoin received by these patients was 1.2 mg/kg/day. Eighteen patients received only one 4-month course of isotretinoin. Fifteen patients received two courses. These included 12 patients with predominantly truncal acne who responded partially to the first course and three patients who had cleared completely after one course of therapy but had mild relapses after an average of six months off of the treatment. All patients were in remission averaging 38 months in duration. Skin biopsies and quantitative measurement of sebum production during therapy indicated a profound inhibition of sebaceous gland size and function, which may be central to the mechanism of action of isotretinoin in acne [70]. Cautions have to been taken that no concurrent topical acne treatment to avoid skin irritation. No concurrent vitamin A supplements or tetracyclines might be used to prevent benign intracranial hypertension.

The medication should also be considered for less severe acne that is resistant to conventional therapy and for those at risk of scarring or psychological morbidity [183,184]. Isotretinoin decreases sebum production, follicular keratinization, and intrafollicular concentration of *P. acnes* [167]. In addition, it has a direct anti-inflammatory effect. The main mechanism is through reducing sebum production by up to 90% (sebopenic). The medication can be used irrespective of age. The recommended daily dosage is 0.5 to 1 mg per kg for 4 to 6 months, starting at 0.5 mg/kg/day to prevent initial flare-up of symptoms, and gradually adjust the dose according to the response [183-186].

Optimal effect can be achieved with higher daily dose. The optimal cumulative dose is 120 mg/kg with minimal post-therapy relapse. Approximately 85% patients report clear of acne after 4 months. Intermittent isotretinoin (0.5 mg/kg/day for 1 week, in every 4 weeks for 6 months) in adults reduces side effects and drug costs but increases rate of relapse (approximately 40%) [185,186]. About 25% of patients may relapse after one treatment. In those cases, a second treatment for another 4 to 6 months may be indicated to obtain desired results. It is often recommended that one lets a few months pass between the two treatments, because the condition can actually improve somewhat in the time after stopping the treatment and waiting a few months also gives the body a chance to recover. Occasionally a third or even a fourth course is used, but the benefits are often less substantial [187,188].

Side effects are dose-related, and include cheilitis, xerosis, conjunctivitis, pruritus, epistaxis, drying of the nasal mucosa, and dry mouth. Other adverse reactions include alopecia, photosensitivity, nausea, vomiting, palmoplantar desquamation, arthralgia, myalgia, delayed wound healing, headache, and increased intracranial pressure. Exacerbation of acne (acne flare-up) may occur in the first month of treatment due to externalization of deep-seated acne. Severe flare-ups may require treatment with oral prednisolone 0.5 to 1 mg/kg/day for 2 to 3 weeks. Prolonged use may cause early epiphyseal closure or hyperostossi. However, no adverse effect was shown on bone mineralization with usual acne course of 4 to 6 months [189]. Laboratory abnormalities associated with the use of isotretinoin include hypertriglyceridemia, hypercholesterolemia, abnormal liver function tests, elevated erythrocyte sedimentation rate, thrombocytosis, anemia and leucopenia [190]. Patient counseling, careful monitoring, and evaluation and management of adverse events are necessary.

The drug has potential teratogenic effects. Women of childbearing age should not be given oral isotretinoin until pregnancy is excluded and an effective form of contraception is being used during treatment and for one month after stopping the medication. Written consent and discussion with parents are required for teenage girls. Two reliable forms of contraception are needed for sexually active girls. In the United States more than 2,000 women became pregnant while taking the drug between 1982 and 2003, with most pregnancies ending in abortion or miscarriage. About 160 babies with birth defects were born [106,191].

There have been concerns about the possible association between isotretinoin therapy and depressive symptoms. An Australian group conducted a prospective study to evaluate depressive symptoms and quality of life in acne patients receiving either isotretinoin or antibiotics/topical treatments. There were 215 patients (mean age 20 years) included in the study. Depression, quality of life and acne severity ratings were assessed at baseline, 1 month, 3 months and end of treatment or 6 months, and compared between both treatment groups. The changes in the mean depression scores did not differ significantly between the two groups (P = 0.62). The incidence of patients treated with isotretinoin who had moderate depressive symptoms remained relatively unchanged from baseline. The changes in the quality-of-life measures scores between treatment groups showed no significant difference. No correlation between isotretinoin dose and depression score was found. Although five patients treated with isotretinoin were withdrawn during the study because of worsening of mood, no definite causal relationship was established. The pilot study does not appear to support any direct link between depression and isotretinoin, apart from being a rare unpredictable idiosyncratic side-effect [192].

Phototherapy

Novel and promising treatments with laser/light devices (such as blue light, red light, pulsed dye laser, infrared lasers, light-emitting diodes, and pulsed light) have been reported to have varying degrees of success in the treatment of acne [193,194]. The main indications are for treating retentional lesions, inflamed lesions, and scars [195]. Studies examining the role of different wavelengths and methods of light treatment have shown that phototherapy with visible light, specifically blue light, has a marked effect on inflammatory acne lesions and seems sufficient for the treatment of acne [193,194]. In addition, the combination of blue-red light radiation seems to be superior to blue light alone, with minimal adverse effects. Photodynamic therapy has also been used, even in nodular and cystic acne, and has excellent therapeutic outcomes, although with significant adverse effects. Recently, low energy pulsed dye laser therapy has been used, and seems to be a promising alternative that would allow the simultaneous treatment of active acne and acne scarring. Some of these studies are summarized as follows according to the year of publication.

Phototherapy has been successfully employed to treat acne - in particular intense ultraviolet light (405 to 420 nm) generated by purpose-built fluorescent lighting, dichroic bulbs, light-emitting diodes (LED) or lasers. Used twice weekly, phototherapy has been shown to reduce the number of acne lesions by about 64%; and is even more effective when applied daily [34]. Presumably, coproporphyrin III that is produced within *P. acnes* generates free radicals when irradiated by ultraviolet light with wavelengths of 407 to 420 nm [35]. These free radicals ultimately kill the bacteria.

Papageorgious et al evaluated the use of blue light (peak at 415 nm) and a mixed blue and red light (peaks at 415 and 660 nm, respectively) in the treatment of acne vulgaris [196]. One hundred and seven patients with mild to moderate acne vulgaris were randomized into four treatment groups: blue light, mixed blue and red light, cool white light and 5% benzoyl peroxide cream. Subjects in the phototherapy groups used portable light sources and irradiation was carried out daily for 15 min. Comparative assessment between the three light sources was made in an observer-blinded fashion, but this could not be achieved for the use of benzoyl peroxide. Assessments were performed every 4 weeks. After 12 weeks of active treatment a mean improvement of 76% (95% CI: 66 to 87) in inflammatory lesions was achieved by the combined blue-red light phototherapy; this was significantly superior to that achieved by blue light (at weeks 4 and 8 but not week 12), benzoyl peroxide (at weeks 8 and 12) or white light (at each assessment). The final mean improvement in comedones by using blue-red light was 58% (95% CI: 45 to 71), again better than that achieved by the other active treatments used, although the differences did not reach significant levels. The authors concluded that phototherapy with mixed blue-red light, probably by combining antibacterial and anti-inflammatory action, is an effective means of treating acne vulgaris of mild to moderate severity, with no significant short-term adverse effects.

Kawada et al treated 30 patients with a high-intensity, enhanced, narrow-band, blue light source and found that phototherapy using this blue light source was effective and well tolerated in acne patients and had an ability to decrease numbers of *P. acnes* [188].

Na et al assessed the efficacy of red light phototherapy with a portable device in acne vulgaris [197]. Twenty-eight volunteers with mild to moderate acne were treated with portable red light-emitting devices in this split-face randomized trial. The right or left side of the face was randomized to treatment side and phototherapy was performed for 15 minutes twice a day for 8 weeks. Clinical photographs, lesion counts, and a visual analog scale were used to assess each side of the face at baseline and weeks 1, 2, 4, and 8, and a split-face comparison was performed. The percent improvement in noninflammatory and inflammatory lesion counts of the treated side was significant compared to the control side (P < 0.005). Visual analog scale decreased from 3.9 to 1.9 on the treatment side and the difference between the treatment and control sides was significant at week 8 (P < 0.005). The study showed that red light phototherapy alone can be a new therapeutic option for acne vulgaris.

Near infrared diode laser low-intensity (soft) phototherapy with the topical application of indocyanine green has been suggested for treatment of acne vulgaris [198]. Twelve volunteers with acne lesions on their faces and/or backs were enrolled in the experiment. Skin areas of the subjects that were 4 x 5 cm^2 were stained with indocyanine green solution for 5 min before laser irradiation (803 nm) at a power density up to 50 mW/cm^2 for 5 to 10 min. For 75% of the subjects, a single treatment was provided and for the other 25%, eight sequential treatments over a period of a month were carried out. Observation a month after the completion of the treatment showed that only the multiple treatments with a combination of indocyanine green and near infrared irradiation reduced inflammation and improved the state of the skin for a month without any side effects. A month after treatment, the improvement was about 80% for the group receiving multiple treatments. Single treatments did not have a prolonged effect

Goldberg et al studied the efficacy phototherapy for acne with a combination of blue and red light [199]. Twenty-four subjects, Fitzpatrick skin types II-V, with symmetric facial acne vulgaris were recruited for the study. Subjects were well matched at baseline in terms of both age and duration of acne. Subjects were treated over eight sessions, two per week 3 days apart, alternating between 415 nm blue light (20 minutes/session, 48 J/cm^2) and 633 nm red light (20 minutes/session, 96 J/cm^2) from a light-emitting diode (LED)-based therapy system. Patients received a mild microdermabrasion before each session. Acne was assessed at baseline and at weeks 2, 4, 8 and 12. Twenty-two patients completed the trial. A mean reduction in lesion count was observed at all follow-up points. At the 4-week follow-up, the mean lesion count reduction was significant at 46% (P = 0.001). At the 12-week follow-up, the mean lesion count reduction was also significant at 81% (P = 0.001). Patient and dermatologist assessments were similar. Severe acne showed a marginally better response than mild acne. Side effects were minimal and transitory. Comedones did not respond to the same extent as inflammatory lesions. The authors concluded that combination blue and red LED therapy is efficacious in the treatment of mild to severe acne, and appears pain- and side effect- free.

Combined blue and red LED phototherapy for acne vulgaris has also been studied [200]. Twenty-four patients with mild to moderately severe facial acne were treated with quasi-monochromatic LED devices, alternating blue (415 nm) and red (633 nm) light. The treatment was performed twice a week for 4 weeks. Objective assays of the skin condition were carried out before and after treatment at each treatment session. Clinical assessments were conducted before treatment, after the 2nd, 4th, and 6th treatment sessions and at 2, 4, and 8 weeks after the final treatment by grading and lesion counting. The final mean percentage improvements in non-inflammatory and inflammatory lesions were 34.28% and 77.93%, respectively. Instrumental measurements indicated that the melanin levels significantly decreased after treatment. Brightened skin tone and improved skin texture were spontaneously reported by 14 patients. The authors concluded that blue and red light combination LED phototherapy is an effective, safe and non-painful treatment for mild to moderately severe acne vulgaris, particularly for papulopustular acne lesions.

In order to study the mechanisms of action of phototherapy, Zane et al exposed 15 women suffering from moderate acne vulgaris of the face to 20 J/cm^2 of broad-band red (lambda: 600 to 750 nm) light twice weekly for 4 weeks [201]. A significant improvement of acne lesions and a significant decrease of skin sebum excretion and transepidermal water loss of the face were registered at the end of the therapy and at the 3-month follow-up visit. The results could be related to a reduced follicular colonization of P. acnes which was lethally damaged by photoactivated endogenous porphyrins. The findings indicated that red light phototherapy may represent an effective, well-tolerated, safe, simple and inexpensive treatment option for moderate acne vulgaris.

Ammad et al evaluated the use of intense blue light within the spectral range of 415 to 425 nm (peak 420 nm) in the treatment of acne vulgaris [202]. Twenty-one patients with mild to moderate facial acne were treated with blue light phototherapy. All patients were given 14-min treatment sessions twice a week for 4 weeks. Acne severity was assessed using the Leeds Technique for grading and lesion counts. Disability was assessed using the Dermatology Life Quality Index (DLQI). In addition, standard digital and cross-polarized light photographs were taken and graded by a blinded evaluator. Visual analog scale scores and cultures for P. acnes were carried out before starting the treatment and upon completion of the treatment. Significant improvement was achieved in the Leeds Acne Grade ($P = 0.001$). The inflammatory ($P = 0.001$) and noninflammatory ($P = 0.06$) lesion counts also improved significantly. A similar change was noted in the DLQI ($P = 0.001$); a degree of significance was also achieved in the patients' and the investigators' visual analog scale scores ($P = 0.01$ and $P = 0.001$, respectively). The authors believed that blue light may be beneficial for the treatment of a select group of mild to moderate acne patients

Photodynamic Therapy

Pollock et al investigated the efficacy of aminolevulinic acid-photodynamic therapy (ALA-PDT) in the treatment of acne and to identify the mode of action, looking specifically at the effects on surface numbers of *P. acnes* and on sebum excretion [113]. Ten patients (nine men and one woman, age range 16 to 40 years) with mild to moderate acne on their backs were recruited. Each patient's back was marked with four 30-cm^2 areas of equal acne severity. Each site was then randomly allocated to either ALA-PDT, light alone, ALA alone or an untreated control site. At baseline, the numbers of inflammatory and noninflammatory acne lesions were counted, sebum excretion measured by Sebutapes (CuDerm, Dallas, TX, U.S.A.) and surface *P. acnes* swabs performed. ALA cream (20% in Unguentum Merck) was applied under occlusion to the ALA-PDT and ALA alone sites for 3 h. Red light from a diode laser was then delivered to the ALA-PDT and light alone sites. Each patient was treated weekly for 3 weeks. Acne lesion counts were performed at each visit. Three weeks following the last treatment, sebum excretion rates and *P. acnes* swabs were repeated. There was a statistically significant reduction in inflammatory acne lesion counts from baseline after the second treatment at the ALA-PDT site but not at any of the other sites. No statistically significant reduction in *P. acnes* numbers or sebum excretion was demonstrated at any sites including the ALA-PDT site. The authors concluded that ALA-PDT is capable of clinically improving acne. An alternative mode of action for ALA-PDT other than direct damage to sebaceous glands or photodynamic killing of *P. acnes* is suggested from the results of this study.

Photodynamic therapy of acne vulgaris using methyl aminolevulinate (MAL-PDT) has also been shown to be an efficient treatment for inflammatory acne [203]. Wiegell et al evaluated the efficacy and tolerability of MAL-PDT in patients with moderate to severe facial acne vulgaris in a randomized, controlled and investigator-blinded trial [203]. Twenty-one patients were assigned to the treatment group and 15 patients to the control group. The treatment group received two MAL-PDT treatments, 2 weeks apart. Both groups were evaluated 4, 8 and 12 weeks after treatment. Twelve weeks after treatment the treatment group showed a 68% reduction from baseline in inflammatory lesions vs. no change in the control group. The authors found no reduction in number of noninflammatory lesions after treatment. All patients experienced moderate to severe pain during treatment and developed severe erythema, pustular eruptions and epithelial exfoliation. Seven patients did not receive the second treatment due to adverse effects.

Laser Treatment

Multiple new lasers and forms of light therapy have been found useful in the treatment of acne. Laser and light treatment act by reacting with the porphyrins produced by *P. acnes* to form unstable and destructive compounds which result in bacterial death [204]. In general, the longer the wavelength of the light is, the deeper is its penetration and thus the greater is its damage to the sebaceous glands. Although blue light is best for the activation of porphyrins, red light is best for deeper penetration and an anti-inflammatory effect. Ultraviolet (UV) light, although it may have anti-inflammatory effects, has been proven to be potentially carcinogenic and have adverse effects such as aging (by UV-A) and burning (by UV-B). Previous studies indicate successful long-term intervention and selective damage of the sebaceous glands by using a diode laser with indocyanine green dye. Mid-infrared lasers have been found to decrease lesion counts while at the same time reduce the oiliness of skin and the scarring process. Nonablative laser treatment of acne scars using the Er:YAG laser with a short-pulsed mode has been successful in reducing the appearance of scars by stimulating neocollagenesis. The light/laser therapy has shown promising results in highly selected patients that require further investigation in greater populations and well-designed protocols

Orringer et al conducted a randomized, single-blind, controlled, split-face clinical trial on a volunteer sample of 40 patients aged 13 years or older with facial acne using pulsed dye laser [205]. Changes in lesion counts from baseline to 12 weeks between treated and untreated sides of the face and in photographic evidence of acne severity as graded by a panel of dermatologists blinded to treatment assignment were compared. After 12 weeks, using intent-to-treat analysis with last observation carried forward, there were no significant differences between laser-treated and untreated skin for changes in mean papule counts (-4.2 vs -2.2; $P = 0.08$), mean pustule counts (0 vs -1.0; $P = 0.12$), or mean comedone counts (2.9 vs 1.6; $P = 0.63$). Grading of serial photographs confirmed the clinical assessments, showing no significant mean (SE) differences in Leeds scores (range, 1 to 12) for treated skin (3.98 [0.32] at baseline and 3.94 [0.27] at week 12) compared with untreated skin (3.83 [0.32] at baseline and 3.79 [0.28] at week 12) (P > 0.99). The study found that the nonpurpuric pulsed dye laser therapy did not result in significant improvement of facial acne and the authors recommended that more research is needed before this laser therapy can be recommended as an acne treatment.

Baugh et al studied the safety and efficacy of the potassium titanyl phosphate (KTP) 532 nm pulsed laser for the treatment of acne vulgaris [206]. Twenty-six subjects, clinically evaluated with moderate facial acne, were enrolled in this single-center prospective trial. The entire facial area for each subject was divided in half and randomly designated as either a treatment or a control side. Each subject was treated with four laser exposures using a KTP 532 nm laser with continuous contact cooling. The results were assessed at 1 and 4 weeks post-final treatment. Primary outcome analysis of the Michaelsson acne severity score demonstrated a mean 34.9% (p = 0.011) and 20.7% (p = 0.25) reduction at the 1-week and 4-week post-final treatments, respectively. Subjective investigator evaluations of overall percent satisfaction indicated that all patients demonstrated a minimum 50% overall satisfaction in treatment outcomes at the 4-week follow-up period. No side effects were encountered. The authors concluded that use of the KTP 532 nm laser for the treatment and management of acne vulgaris is safe, effective, and with results enduring up to 4 weeks post-treatment

In order to observe the therapeutic effects of He-Ne laser auricular irradiation plus body acupuncture for acne vulgaris, 68 cases of acne vulgaris were randomly divided into a treatment group of 36 cases treated with He-Ne laser auricular irradiation plus body acupuncture, and a control group of 32 cases treated with body acupuncture only. The results showed that the cure rate was 77.8% in the treatment group and 46.9% in the control group (P < 0.05), indicating that He-Ne laser auricular irradiation plus body acupuncture may exhibit better effects for acne vulgaris [207].

Sami et al evaluated the effectiveness of pulsed dye laser (PDL), intense pulsed light (IPL) and LED phototherapy for the treatment of moderate to severe acne vulgaris [208]. They randomly divided 45 patients with moderate to severe acne into 3 equal groups. Group 1 was treated with a PDL, group 2 was treated with IPL, and group 3 was treated with a blue-red combination LED. Treatment was continued until a ≥ 90% clearance of patient lesions was achieved. Clinical assessments were conducted before starting treatment, at 1 month as a midpoint evaluation, and after the final treatment session. The authors found that patients treated with the PDL reached a ≥ 90% clearance of their inflammatory lesions after a mean of 4.1 ± 1.39 sessions, while patients treated with IPL required a mean of 6 ± 2.05 sessions. Patients treated with the LED required a mean of 10 ± 3.34 sessions. At the mid-point evaluation, the percent reduction in acne lesions treated with the PDL was 90% or more, in cases of IPL and the LED, the percent reductions were 41.7% and 35.3%, respectively. Laser and light phototherapy sessions were well tolerated with minimal adverse events experienced as being mild and usually self-limiting. The authors concluded that laser and light phototherapy was useful therapeutic option for treatment of moderate to severe acne.

Miscellaneous Treatments

Occasionally, comdone extraction is used to provide an immediate cosmetic effect. Comedone extraction, if improperly performed, may result in rupture of the pilosebaceous duct leading to the production of inflammatory papules and an actual worsening of appearance.

Several physical modalities are helpful in management of scars resulting from acne. Chemical peels can be used to treat superficial scars and hyperpigmentation, preferably after acne has been brought under control [14]. Trichloacetic acid, alpha hydroxyl acid, and salicylic acid have been used with success in this regard. Dermabrasion or laserbrasion can help in treating superficial scars if carried out carefully. Complications of dermabrasion include infection, erythema, hypertrophic scars, and pigmentary alterations. Deeper scars can be smoothed by collagen implantation. Zyderm, a highly purified, non-antigenic bovine collagen homogenate, can be injected intradermally to restore even surface contours. Adverse reactions are occasionally encountered and include itching and pain at the injection site, erythema, induration, arthralgia, and local granuloma formation. Nonablative laser modalities have shown some potential for the treatment of atrophic, sclerotic, and pitted acne scars.

Topical steroids have been used for the treatment of cystic acne or keloid. Topical clobetasol proprionate can be applied twice daily for 5 days for the treatment of cystic acne. Intralesional injection of triamcinolone acetonide (Kenalog), 1.0 to 2.5 mg per mL of solution, will lead to rapid resolution of most cystic lesions in two to three days [209]. The corticosteroid is injected into the cyst with a 27- to 30-gauge needle. It is important to inject a minimal amount and to do so superficially to avoid local steroid atrophy. Side effects are minimal, but may include a temporary whitening of the skin around the injection point; and occasionally a small depression forms, which may persist, although often fills eventually. This method also carries a much smaller risk of scarring than surgical removal. Intralesional triamcinolone injection has also been used for the treatment of keloid.

A number of less widely used treatments have been used. Descriptions and studies on their efficacy are scanty. There are treatments for acne using herbs such as aloe vera, Neem Haldi (Turmeric) and Papaya [36]. There is limited evidence from medical studies on some of these products, although others have been proven effective. Products from Rubia cordifolia, Curcuma longa (commonly known as Turmeric), Hemidesmus indicus (known as ananthamoola or anantmula), and Azadirachta indica (Neem) have been shown to have anti-inflammatory effects, but not aloe vera [36].

Nicotinamide, (Vitamin B_3) used topically in the form of a gel, was shown to be more effective than a topical antibiotic used for the treatment of acne, as well as having fewer side effects in the study by Shalita et al [210]. Topical nicotinamide is available both on prescription and over-the-counter. The property of topical nicotinamide's benefit in treating acne seems to be its anti-inflammatory nature. It is also purported to result in increased synthesis of collagen, keratin, involucrin and flaggrin. However, latter studies have not found the addition of nicotinamide useful. A total of 75 patients with inflammatory acne vulgaris were divided into three groups [211]. Group A (treatment-naïve patients) was treated with a combination of 4% nicotinamide and 1% clindamycin, group B (treatment-naïve) was treated with plain 1% clindamycin and group C (resistant cases who did not respond satisfactorily to topical antibiotics) was also treated with the combination of 4% nicotinamide and 1% clindamycin. At the end of 8 weeks the results were compared. It was concluded that nicotinamide had no added benefit in inflammatory or resistant acne [211,212].

Tea tree oil (melaleuca oil) dissolved in a carrier (5% strength) has been used with some success, where it is comparable to benzoyl peroxide but without excessive drying [36]. Orally administered zinc gluconate has been shown to be effective in the treatment of inflammatory acne, although less so than tetracyclines [145,213]. In a double-blind trial using low doses of zinc gluconate for inflammatory acne, Dreno et al obtained a significantly different result between zinc and placebo groups in the inflammatory score (p less than 0.02). This efficiency could be explained by the action of zinc on inflammatory cells, especially granulocytes [213]. The investigators further performed multi-center randomized comparative double-blind controlled clinical trial of the safety and efficacy of zinc gluconate versus minocycline hydrochloride in the treatment of inflammatory acne vulgaris [145]. Three hundred thirty two patients received either 30 mg elemental zinc or 100 mg minocycline over 3 months. The primary endpoint was defined as the percentage of the clinical success rate on day 90 (i.e. more than 2/3 decrease in inflammatory lesions, i.e. papules and pustules). This clinical success rate was 31.2% for zinc and 63.4% for minocycline. Minocycline nevertheless showed a 9% superiority in action at 1 month and 17% at 3 months, with respect to the mean change in lesion count. The authors concluded that minocycline and zinc gluconate are both effective in the treatment of inflammatory acne, but minocycline has a superior effect evaluated to be 17% in our study.

Sodium ascorbyl phosphate represents a stable precursor of vitamin C that ensures a constant delivery of vitamin C into the skin. Klock et al showed that 1% sodium ascorbyl phosphate has a strong antimicrobial effect on *P. acnes* in a time-kill study [214]. In a human *in vivo* study involving 20 subjects, Klock et al showed that a sodium ascorbyl phosphate O/W formulation significantly prevented the UVA-induced sebum oxidation up to 40%. Subsequently, Klock et al performed an open *in vivo* study with 60 subjects with a 5% sodium ascorbyl phosphate lotion over 12 weeks. The efficacy ranked as excellent and good of SAP was 76.9%, which was superior compared with a widely prescribed acne treatment. The authors concluded that sodium ascorbyl phosphate is efficient in the prevention and treatment of acne vulgaris. Sodium ascorbyl phosphate can be used in a non-antibiotic and effective treatment or co-treatment of acne with no side effects.

Chapter 10

FUTURE DEVELOPMENTS

Responses to *P. acnes* by host immunity play important roles in its pathogenesis, and identifying immune modulators that attenuate inflammatory responses against *P. acnes* and the inhibition of bacterial growth may lead to novel avenues of immunologic intervention [215]. Vaccination appears a logical treatment. However, there have been no acne vaccines for humans to date. A vaccine against inflammatory acne has been tested successfully in mice, but it is not certain that it would work similarly in humans [187]. A 2007 microbiology article reporting the first genome sequencing of a *P. acnes* bacteriophage (PA6) said this "should greatly enhance the development of a potential bacteriophage therapy to treat acne and therefore overcome the significant problems associated with long-term antibiotic therapy and bacterial resistance" [215].

New developments and future trends represent low-dose long-term isotretinoin regimens, new isotretinoin formulations (micronized isotretinoin), isotretinoin metabolites, combination treatments to reduce toxicity, insulin-sensitizing agents, 5 α-reductase type 1 inhibitors, antisense oligonucleotide molecules, and, especially, new anti-inflammatory agents, such as lipoxygenase inhibitors [216].

Chapter 11

PROGNOSIS

The natural course of mild acne usually lasts for 5 years or less. Severe acne may last more than 10 years in some cases, and 95% of all acne patients suffer some degree of facial scarring [217]. Early onset acne predicts subsequent severe acne and scarring [183,218]. Other risk factors for scarring include nodular acne, late commencement of treatment, inflamed lesions, and truncal acne in the male [217].

Prognosis of infantile acne is generally good [76]. In a retrospective review of 29 patients (24 boys and five girls) with infantile acne, no infants had any clinically obvious endocrinopathy [76]. Patients with mild acne responded well to topical treatment (benzoyl peroxide, erythromycin and retinoids). All but two infants with moderate acne responded well to oral erythromycin 125 mg twice daily and topical therapy. Patients with erythromycin-resistant *P. acnes* required trimethoprim 100 mg twice daily. Most patients were able to stop oral antibiotics within 18 months. In 38% of children, long-term oral antibiotics (> 24 months) were required. The time for clearance of the acne was 6 to 40 months (median 18). One patient required oral isotretinoin that cleared the acne in 4 months. Five patients (17%) were left with scarring. Treatment is similar to that of adult acne, with the exclusion of the use of tetracyclines. When necessary, oral isotretinoin can be used. There appears to be a trend towards higher incidence and greater severity of acne vulgaris in teenage years in patients with a history of infantile acne compared to their peers [12].

Although the prognosis of acne is generally good, the psychosocial consequences such as anxiety, depression, loss of social esteem [219,220], employment difficulties, emotional, social and psychological disability are similar to patients with chronic disabling such as asthma, epilepsy, diabetes, back pain or arthritis [184].

SUMMARY

Acne is a highly prevalent, chronic inflammatory disease of pilosebaceous units. Pathogenic factors include increased production of sebum, proliferation of *P. acnes* with resultant increase in chemotactic factors and proinflammatory mediators which lead to inflammation, release of lipids into the sebaceous duct and follicle, and obstruction of the pilosebaceous canal caused by hyperproliferation and shedding of keratinocytes in clumps. Acne lesions tend to occur on the face, and to a lesser extent, on the upper back. Acne can be psychologically traumatic and can severely compromise quality of life.

For mild acne, a combination topical treatment such as benzoyl peroxide ± erythromycin or tretinoin is advocated [129]. The patient should be reviewed in 3 months. For moderate acne, especially when acne scars start to occur, or if above fails, an oral antibiotic, depending on cost and side effects, will be used, switching to alternative antibiotic if no improvement in 3 months. Antibiotics with anti-inflammatory properties, such as tetracyclines (oxytetracycline, tetracycline chloride, doxycycline, minocycline and limecycline) and macrolide antibiotics (erythromycin and azithromycin) are the agents of choice for papulopustular acne, even though the emerging resistant bacterial strains are minimizing their effect, especially regarding erythromycin. Systemic antibiotics should be administered during a period of 8 to 12 weeks. Topical therapy should be continued during the course of oral antibiotic therapy and afterwards for a number of years. Dissimilar oral and topical antibiotics should be avoided if possible to prevent antibiotic resistance. In severe papulopustular and in nodulocystic/conglobate acne, oral isotretinoin is the treatment of choice. The drug is extremely effective but repeat courses may be necessary. Hormonal treatment represents an alternative regimen in female acne, whereas it is mandatory in resistant, severe pubertal or post-adolescent forms of the disease. Low-dose corticosteroids (prednisone, prednisolone, or dexamethasone) are indicated in patients with adrenal hyperandrogenism or acne fulminans.

In infantile acne, treatment options include benzoyl 2.5% gel, topical erythromycin, tretinoin 0.01% cream for comedones, oral erythromycin for inflammed papules (oral trimethoprim if resistant to erythromycin), or oral isotretinoin if acne is severe or resistant [221-223]. The dose of isotretinoin used ranges from 0.2 mg/kg/day to 1.5 mg/kg/day and the treatment duration varies from 5 to 14 months [223].

REFERENCES

[1] McInturff, JE; Kim, J. The role of toll-like receptors in the pathophysiology of acne. *Semin. Cutan. Med. Surg.* 2005; 24:73-78.

[2] Goodman, G. Acne and acne scarring - the case for active and early intervention. *Aust. Fam. Physician.* 2006; 35:503-504.

[3] Purvis, D. Acne, anxiety, depression and suicide in teenagers: A cross-sectional survey of New Zealand secondary school students. *J. Paediatr. Child Health* 2006; 42:793-796.

[4] Picardi, AM; Mazzotti, ED; Pasquini, PMM. Prevalence and correlates of suicidal ideation among patients with skin disease. *J. Am. Acad. Dermatol.* 2006; 54:420-426.

[5] Krowchuk, DP; Lucky, AW. Managing adolescent acne. *Adolesc. Med.* 2001; 12:355-374.

[6] Ballanger, F; Baudry, P; N'Guyen, JM; et al. Heredity: a prognostic factor for acne. *Dermatology.* 2006. 212:145-149.

[7] Taylor, SC; Cook-Bolden, F; Rahman, Z; et al. Acne vulgaris in skin of color. *J. Am. Acad. Dermatol.* 2002; 46(Suppl 2):S98-S106.

[8] Kilkenny, M; Merlin, K; Plunkett, A; et al. The prevalence of common skin conditions in Australian school students: 3. acne vulgaris. *Br. J. Dermatol.* 1998; 139:840-845.

[9] Cordain, L; Lindeberg, S; Hurtado, M; et al. Acne vulgaris: a disease of Western civilization. *Arch..Dermatol.* 2002; 138:1584-1590.

[10] Wu, TQ; Mei, SQ; Zhang, JX; et al. Prevalence and risk factors of facial acne vulgaris among Chinese adolescents. *Int. J. Adoles. Med. Health.* 2007; 19:407-412.

[11]   Freyre, EA; Rebaza, RM; Sami, DA; et al. The prevalence of facial acne in Peruvian adolescents and its relation to their ethnicity. *J. Adoles.Health.* 1998; 22:480-484.

[12]   Chew, EW; Bingham, A; Burrows, D. Incidence of acne vulgaris in patients with infantile acne. *Clin. Exp. Dermatol.* 1990; 15:376-377.

[13]   Bergfeld, WF. The pathophysiology of acne vulgaris in children and adolescents, Part 1. *Cutis.* 2004; 74:92-97.

[14]   Leung, AK; Robson, WL. Acne. *J. R. Soc. Health.* 1991; 111:57-60.

[15]   Holmes, RL; Williams, M; Cunliffe, WJ. Pilo-sebaceous duct obstruction and acne. *Br. J. Dermatol.* 1972; 87:327-332.

[16]   Borelli, C; Plewig, G; Degitz K. Pathophysiology of acne. *Hautarzt.* 2005; 56:1013-1017.

[17]   Webster, GF. The pathophysiology of acne. *Cutis.* 2005; 76(Suppl 2):4-7.

[18]   Bergfeld, WF. The pathophysiology of acne vulgaris in children and adolescents, part 2: tailoring treatment. *Cutis.* 2004; 74:189-192.

[19]   Cunliffe, WJ; Holland, DB; Jeremy, A. Comedone formation: etiology, clinical presentation, and treatment. *Clin. Dermatol.* 2004; 22:367-374.

[20]   Arbesman, H. Dairy and acne--the iodine connection. *J. Am. Acad. Dermatol.* 2005; 53:1102.

[21]   Leyden, JJ. McGinley KJ, Mills, OH; et al. Propionibacterium levels in patients with and without acne vulgaris. *J. Invest. Dermatol.* 1975; 65:382-384.

[22]   Jeremy, AH; Holland, DB; Roberts, SG; et al. Inflammatory events are involved in acne lesion initiation. *J. Invest. Dermatol.* 2003; 121:20-27.

[23]   Cunliffe, WJ; Holland, DB; Clark, SM; et al. Comedogenesis: some aetiological, clinical and therapeutic strategies. *Dermatology.* 2003; 206:11-16.

[24]   James, WD. Clinical practice. Acne. *N. Engl. J. Med.* 2005; 352:1463-1472.

[25]   Kang, BS; Seo, JG; Lee, GS; et al. Antimicrobial activity of enterocins from Enterococcus faecalis SL-5 against Propionibacterium acnes, the causative agent in acne vulgaris, and its therapeutic effect. *J. Microbiol.* 2009; 47:101-109.

[26]   Nakatsuji, T; Shi, Y; Zhu, W; et al. Bioengineering a humanized acne microenvironment model: proteomics analysis of host responses to Propionibacterium acnes infection in vivo. *Proteomics.* 2008; 8:3406-3415.

[27] Oprica, C; Emtestam, L; Lapins, J; et al. Antibiotic-resistant Propionibacterium acnes on the skin of patients with moderate to severe acne in Stockholm. *Anaerobe.* 2004; 10:155-164.

[28] Wilcox, HE; Farrar, MD; Cunliffe, WJ; et al E. Resolution of inflammatory acne vulgaris may involve regulation of CD4+ T-cell responses to Propionibacterium acnes. *Br. J. Dermatol.* 2007; 156:460-465.

[29] Gubelin, W; Martinez, MA; Molina, MT; et al. Antimicrobial susceptibility of strains of Propionibacterium acnes isolated from inflammatory acne. *Rev. Latinoam. Microbiol.* 2006; 48:14-16.

[30] Dreno, B; Foulc, P; Reynaud, A; et al. Effect of zinc gluconate on propionibacterium acnes resistance to erythromycin in patients with inflammatory acne: in vitro and in vivo study. *Eur. J. Dermatol.* 2005; 15:152-155.

[31] Bojar, RA; Holland, KT. Acne and Propionibacterium acnes. *Clin. Dermatol.* 2004; 22:375-379.

[32] Tan, HH; Goh, CL; Yeo, MG; et al. Antibiotic sensitivity of Propionibacterium acnes isolates from patients with acne vulgaris in a tertiary dermatological referral centre in Singapore. *Ann. Acad. Med. Singapore.* 2001; 30:22-25.

[33] Farrar, MD; Howson, KM; Bojar, RA; et al. Genome sequence and analysis of a Propionibacterium acnes bacteriophage. *J. Bacteriol.* 2007; 4161-4167.

[34] Kjeldstad, B. Photoinactivation of Propionibacterium acnes by near-ultraviolet light. *Z. Naturforsch.* 1984; 39:300-302.

[35] Ashkenazi, H; Malik, Z; Harth, Y; et al. Eradication of Propionibacterium acnes by its endogenic porphyrins after illumination with high intensity blue light. *FEMS. Immunol. Med. Microbiol.* 2003; 35:17-24.

[36] Jain, A; Basal, E. Inhibition of Propionibacterium acnes-induced mediators of inflammation by Indian herbs. *Phytomedicine.* 2003; 10:34-38.

[37] Farrar, MD; Ingham, E. Acne: inflammation. *Clin. Dermatol.* 2004; 22:380-384.

[38] Akamatsu, H; Horio, T. The possible role of reactive oxygen species generated by neutrophils in mediating acne inflammation. *Dermatology.* 1998; 196:82-85.

[39] Akamatsu, H; Horio, T; Hattori K. Increased hydrogen peroxide generation by neutrophils from patients with acne inflammation. *Int. J. Dermatol.* 2003; 42:366-369.

[40] Toyoda, M; Morohashi, M. New aspects in acne inflammation. *Dermatology.* 2003; 206:17-23.

[41] Zouboulis, CC. Acne and sebaceous gland function. *Clin. Dermatol.* 2004; 22:360-366.

[42] Deplewski, D; Rosenfield, RL. Role of hormones in pilosebaceous unit development. *Endocrin. Rev.* 2000; 21:363-392.

[43] Thiboutotn, D. Acne: hormonal concepts and therapy. *Clin. Dermatol.* 2004; 22:419-428.

[44] Schafern, T; Nienhausn, A; Vielufn, D; et al. Epidemiology of acne in the general population: the risk of smoking. *Br. J. Dermatol.* 2001; 145:100-104.

[45] Stoll, S; Shalita, AR; Webster, GF; et. The effect of the menstrual cycle on acne. *J. Am. Acad. Dermatol.* 2001; 45:957-960.

[46] Anderson, PC. Foods as the cause of acne. *Am. Fam. Physician.* 1971; 3:102-103.

[47] Fries, JH. Chocolate: a review of published reports of allergic and other deleterious effects, real or presumed. *Ann. Allergy.* 1978; 41:195-207.

[48] Wolf, R; Matz, H; Orion, E. Acne and diet. *Clin. Dermatol.* 2004; 22:387-393.

[49] Cordain, L. Implications for the role of diet in acne. *Semin. Cutan. Med.Surg.* 2005; 24:84-91.

[50] Webster, GF. Commentary: diet and acne. *J. Am. Acad..Dermatol.* 2008; 58:794-795.

[51] Adebamowo, CA; Spiegelman, D; Danby, FW; et al. High school dietary dairy intake and teenage acne. *J. Am. Acad. Dermatol.* 2005; 52:207-214.

[52] Adebamowo, CA; Spiegelman, D; Berkey, CS; et al. Milk consumption and acne in adolescent girls. *Dermatol. Online J.* 2006; 12:1.

[53] Adebamowo, CA; Spiegelman, D; Berkey, CS; Danby, FW; et al. Milk consumption and acne in teenaged boys. *J. Am. Acad. Dermatol.* 2008; 58:787-793.

[54] Fulton, JE Jr.; Plewig, G; Kligman, AM. Effect of chocolate on acne vulgaris. *JAMA.* 1969; 210:2071-2074.

[55] Danby, FW. Diet and acne. *Clin. Dermatol.* 2008; 26:93-96.

[56] Smith, R; Mann, N; Makelainen, H; et al. A pilot study to determine the short-term effects of a low glycemic load diet on hormonal markers of

acne: a nonrandomized, parallel, controlled feeding trial. *Mol. Nutrit. Food Res.* 2008; 52:718-726.

[57] Smith, RN; Mann, NJ; Braue, A; et al. The effect of a high-protein, low glycemic-load diet versus a conventional, high glycemic-load diet on biochemical parameters associated with acne vulgaris: a randomized, investigator-masked, controlled trial. *J. Am. Acad. Dermatol.* 2007; 57:247-256.

[58] Selva, DM; Hogeveen, KN; Innis, SM; et al. Monosaccharide-induced lipogenesis regulates the human hepatic sex hormone-binding globulin gene. *J. Clin. Invest.* 2007; 117:3979-3987.

[59] Aizawa, H; Niimura, M. Elevated serum insulin-like growth factor-1 (IGF-1) levels in women with postadolescent acne. *J. Dermatol.* 1995; 22:249-252.

[60] Cappel, M; Mauger, D; Thiboutot, D. Correlation between serum levels of insulin-like growth factor 1, dehydroepiandrosterone sulfate, and dihydrotestosterone and acne lesion counts in adult women. *Arch. Dermatol.* 2005; 141:333-338.

[61] Aizawa, H; Niimura, M. Mild insulin resistance during oral glucose tolerance test (OGTT) in women with acne. *J. Dermatol.* 1996; 23:526-529.

[62] Fleischer, AB Jr.; Feldman, SR; Bradham, DD. Office-based physician services provided by dermatologists in the United States in 1990. *J. Invest.Dermatol.* 1994; 102:93-97.

[63] Smith, RN; Mann, NJ; Braue, A; et al. A low-glycemic-load diet improves symptoms in acne vulgaris patients: a randomized controlled trial. *Am. J. Clin. Nutrit.* 2007; 86:107-115.

[64] Smith, RN; Braue, A; Varigos, GA; et al. The effect of a low glycemic load diet on acne vulgaris and the fatty acid composition of skin surface triglycerides. *J. Dermatolog. Sci.* 2008; 50:41-52.

[65] El Akawi, Z; Abdel-Latif, N; Abdul-Razzak, K. Does the plasma level of vitamins A and E affect acne condition? *Clin. Exp. Dermatol.* 2006; 31:430-434.

[66] Magin, P; Pond, D; Smith, W; et al. A systematic review of the evidence for 'myths and misconceptions' in acne management: diet, face-washing and sunlight. *Fam. Pract.* 2005; 22:62-70.

[67] Wuthrich, B; Much, T. Acne vulgaris: results of food allergen tests and a controlled elimination diet (author's transl). *Dermatologica.* 1978; 157:294-295.

[68] Shalita, AR. Acne: clinical presentations. *Clin. Dermatol.* 2004; 22:385-386.

[69] Krakowski, AC; Eichenfield, LF. Pediatric acne: clinical presentations, evaluation, and management. *J. Drugs Dermatol.* 2007; 6:589-593.

[70] Peck, GL; Olsen, TG; Butkus, D; et al. Isotretinoin versus placebo in the treatment of cystic acne. A randomized double-blind study. *J. Am. Acad. Dermatol.* 1982; 6(4 Pt 2 Suppl):735-745.

[71] Karvonen, SL. Acne fulminans: report of clinical findings and treatment of twenty-four patients. *J. Am. Acad. Dermatol.* 1993; 28:572-579.

[72] Laasonen, LS; Karvonen, SL; Reunala, TL. Bone disease in adolescents with acne fulminans and severe cystic acne: radiologic and scintigraphic findings. *Am. J. Roentgenol.* 1994; 162:1161-1165.

[73] Stankler, L; Campbell, AG. Neonatal acne vulgaris: a possible feature of the fetal hydantoin syndrome. *Br. J. Dermatol.* 1980; 103:453-455.

[74] Feldman, S; Careccia, RE; Barham, KL; et al. Diagnosis and treatment of acne. *Am. Fam. Physician.* 2004; 69:2123-2130.

[75] Lucky, AW. A review of infantile and pediatric acne. *Dermatology.* 1998; 196:95-97.

[76] Cunliffe, WJ; Baron, SE; Coulson, IH. A clinical and therapeutic study of 29 patients with infantile acne. *Br. J. Dermatol.* 2001; 145:463-466.

[77] MacFarlane, JT; Davies, D. Management of hereditary angio-oedema with low-dose danazol. *Br. Med. J. (Clin. Res. Ed.)* 1981; 282:1275.

[78] Goulden, V; Clark, SM; Cunliffe, WJ. Post-adolescent acne: a review of clinical features. *Br. J. Dermatol.* 1997; 136:66-70.

[79] Diamanti-Kandarakis, E. Current aspects of antiandrogen therapy in women. *Curr. Pharmaceut. Design.* 1999; 5:707-723.

[80] Shalita, AR. Lipid and teratogenic effects of retinoids. *J. Am. Acad. Dermatol.* 1988; 19:197-198.

[81] Krowchuk, DP; Stancin, T; Keskinen, R; et al. The psychosocial effects of acne on adolescents. *Pediatr. Dermatol.* 1991; 8:332-338.

[82] Witkowski, JA; Parish, LC. The assessment of acne: an evaluation of grading and lesion counting in the measurement of acne. *Clin. Dermatol.* 2004; 22:394-397.

[83] Burke, BM; Cunliffe, WJ. The assessment of acne vulgaris--the Leeds technique. *Br. J. Dermatol.* 1984; 111:83-92.

[84] Allen, BS; Smith, JG Jr. Various parameters for grading acne vulgaris. *Arch. Dermatol.* 1982; 118(1):23-25.

[85] Fehnel, SE; McLeod, LD; Brandman, J; et al. Responsiveness of the Acne-Specific Quality of Life Questionnaire (Acne-QoL) to treatment

for acne vulgaris in placebo-controlled clinical trials. *Qual. Life Res.* 2002; 11:809-816.

[86] Henkel, V; Moehrenschlager, M; Hegerl, U; et al. Screening for depression in adult acne vulgaris patients: tools for the dermatologist. *J. Cos. Dermatol.* 2002; 1:202-207.

[87] Thiboutot, DM. Hormonal therapy of acne. *Dermatol. Ther.* 1998;6:39-43.

[88] Jemec, GB; Jemec, B. Acne: treatment of scars. *Clin. Dermatol.* 2004; 22:434-438.

[89] Cunliffe, WJ. Acne and unemployment. *Br. J. Dermatol.* 1986; 115:386.

[90] Thiboutot, DM. An overview of acne and its treatment. *Cutis.* 1996; 57(Suppl 1):8-12.

[91] Thiboutot, DM. Overview of acne and its treatment. *Cutis.* 2008; 81(Suppl 1):3-7.

[92] Boni, R; Hafner, J; Krasovec, M. Acne and its treatment possibilities. *Schweiz. Med. Wochenschr.* 1999; 129:1496-1503.

[93] Rodondi, N; Darioli, R; Ramelet, AA; et al. High risk for hyperlipidemia and the metabolic syndrome after an episode of hypertriglyceridemia during 13-cis retinoic acid therapy for acne: a pharmacogenetic study. *Ann. Int. Med.* 2002; 136:582-589.

[94] Ott, F; Bollag, W; Geiger, JM. Oral 9-cis-retinoic acid versus 13-cis-retinoic acid in acne therapy. *Dermatology.* 1996; 193:124-126.

[95] Egger, SF; Huber-Spitzy, V; Bohler, K; et al. Ocular side effects associated with 13-cis-retinoic acid therapy for acne vulgaris: clinical features, alterations of tearfilm and conjunctival flora. *Acta Ophthalmol. Scand.* 1995; 73:355-357.

[96] Sitzmann, JH; Bauer, FW; Cunliffe, WJ; et al. In situ hybridization analysis of CRABP II expression in sebaceous follicles from 13-cis retinoic acid-treated acne patients. *Br. J. Dermatol.* 1995; 133:241-248.

[97] Boudou, P; Chivot, M; Vexiau, P; et al. Evidence for decreased androgen 5 alpha-reduction in skin and liver of men with severe acne after 13-cis-retinoic acid treatment. *J. Clin. Endocrinol. Metab.* 1994; 78:1064-1069.

[98] Perkins, W; Crocket, KV; Hodgins, MB; et al. The effect of treatment with 13-cis-retinoic acid on the metabolic burst of peripheral blood neutrophils from patients with acne. *Br. J. Dermatol.* 1991; 124:429-432.

[99] Poljacki, M; Duran, V; Stojanovic, S. Personal experience with the use of 13-cis-retinoic acid in the therapy of severe forms of acne vulgaris. *Med. Pregled.* 1990; 43(3-4):156-158.

[100] Plewig, G; Hennes, R; Maas, B; et al. Remission behavior following low-dose 13-cis-retinoic acid in papulopustular acne. *Z. Hautkr.* 1986; 61:1205-1210.

[101] Langner, A; Wolska, H; Fraczykowska, M; et al. 13-cis-Retinoic acid and tetracycline versus 13-cis-retinoic acid alone in the treatment of nodulocystic acne. *Dermatologica.* 1985; 170:185-188.

[102] Corlin, R; Maas, B; Mack-Hennes, A. 13-cis-retinoic acid. Low dosage oral use in acne papulopustulosa. Results of a multicenter study. *Hautarzt.* 1984; 35:623-629.

[103] Hennes, R; Mack, A; Schell, H; et al. 13-cis-retinoic acid in conglobate acne. A follow-up study of 14 trial centers. *Arch. Dermatol. Res.* 1984; 276:209-215.

[104] Meigel, W; Gollnick, H; Wokalek, H; et al. Oral treatment of acne conglobata using 13-cis-retinoic acid. Results of the German multicentric study following 24 weeks of treatment. *Hautarzt.* 1983; 34:387-397.

[105] Stewart, ME; Benoit, AM; Stranieri, AM; et al. Effect of oral 13-cis-retinoic acid at three dose levels on sustainable rates of sebum secretion and on acne. *J. Am. Acad. Dermatol.* 1983; 8:532-538.

[106] Jones, H; Blanc, D; Cunliffe, WJ. 13-cis retinoic acid and acne. *Lancet.* 1980; 2:1048-1049.

[107] Krowchuk, DP. Managing acne in adolescents. *Pediatr. Clin. North Am.* 2000; 47:841-857.

[108] Webster, GF. Acne vulgaris. *BMJ.* 2002; 325:475-479.

[109] Gollnick, H; Cunliffe, W; Berson, D; et al. Management of acne: a report from a Global Alliance to Improve Outcomes in Acne. *J. Am. Acad. Dermatol.* 2003; 49(1 Suppl):S1-37.

[110] Rigopoulos, D; Ioannides, D; Kalogeromitros, D; et al. Comparison of topical retinoids in the treatment of acne. *Clin. Dermatol.* 2004; 22:408-411.

[111] Katsambas, AD; Stefanaki, C; Cunliffe, WJ. Guidelines for treating acne. *Clin. Dermatol.* 2004; 22:439-444.

[112] Gollnick, HP; Graupe, K; Zaumseil, RP. [Azelaic acid 15% gel in the treatment of acne vulgaris. Combined results of two double-blind clinical comparative studies]. *J. Deuts. Dermatol. Ges.* 2004; 2:841-847.

[113] Pollock, B; Turner, D; Stringer, MR; et al. Topical aminolaevulinic acid-photodynamic therapy for the treatment of acne vulgaris: a study of clinical efficacy and mechanism of action. *Br. J. Dermatol.* 2004; 151:616-622.

[114] Haider, A; Shaw, JC. Treatment of acne vulgaris. *JAMA.* 2004; 292:726-735.

[115] Katsambas, AD. RALGA (Diacneal), a retinaldehyde and glycolic acid association and postinflammatory hyperpigmentation in acne - a review. *Dermatology.* 2005; 210 (Suppl 1):39-45.

[116] Sinclair, W; Jordaan, HF; Global Alliance to Improve Outcomes in Acne. Acne guideline 2005 update. *S. Afr. Med. J.* 2005; 95:881-892.

[117] Zaenglein, AL; Thiboutot, DM. Expert committee recommendations for acne management. *Pediatrics.* 2006; 118:1188-1199.

[118] Ochsendorf, FR; Degitz K. Drug therapy of acne. *Hautarzt.* 2008; 59:579-589.

[119] Purdy, S; de Berker, D. Acne. *BMJ.* 2006; 333:949-953.

[120] Strauss, JS; Krowchuk, DP; Leyden, JJ; et al. Guidelines of care for acne vulgaris management. *J. Am. Acad.Dermatol.* 2007; 56:651-663.

[121] Shalita, AR. Clinical aspects of acne. *Dermatology.* 1998; 196:93-94.

[122] Lucky, AW; Leach, AD; Laskarzewski, P; et al. Use of an emollient as a steroid-sparing agent in the treatment of mild to moderate atopic dermatitis in children. *Pediatr. Dermatol.* 1997; 14:321-324.

[123] Holland, DB; Jeremy, AH; Roberts, SG; et al. Inflammation in acne scarring: a comparison of the responses in lesions from patients prone and not prone to scar. *Br. J. Dermatol.* 2004; 150:72-81.

[124] Holland, DB; Jeremy, AH. The role of inflammation in the pathogenesis of acne and acne scarring. Semin. *Cutan. Med. Surg.* 2005; 24:79-83.

[125] Webster, GF; Guenther, L; Poulin, YP; et al. A multicenter, double-blind, randomized comparison study of the efficacy and tolerability of once-daily tazarotene 0.1% gel and adapalene 0.1% gel for the treatment of facial acne vulgaris. *Cutis.* 2002; 69(Suppl 2):4-11.

[126] Katsambas, A; Papakonstantinou, A. Acne: systemic treatment. *Clin. Dermatol.* 2004; 22:412-418.

[127] Krautheim, A; Gollnick, HP. Acne: topical treatment. *Clin. Dermatol.* 2004; 22:398-407.

[128] Cunliffe, WJ; Holland, DB; Clark, SM; et al. Comedogenesis: some new aetiological, clinical and therapeutic strategies. *Br. J. Dermatol.* 2000; 142:1084-1091.

[129] Olsen, TG. Therapy of acne. *Med. Clin. North Am.* 1982; 66:851-871.

[130] Chalker, DK; Shalita, A; Smith, JG; et al. A double-blind study of the effectiveness of a 3% erythromycin and 5% benzoyl peroxide combination in the treatment of acne vulgaris. *J. Am. Acad. Dermatol.* 1983; 9:933-936.

[131] Burke, B; Eady, EA; Cunliffe, WJ. Benzoyl peroxide versus topical erythromycin in the treatment of acne vulgaris. *Br. J. Dermatol.* 1983; 108:199-204.

[132] Webster, GM. Combination azelaic acid therapy for acne vulgaris. *J. Am. Acad. Dermatol.* 2000; 43:S47-S50.

[133] Hirschmann, JV. Topical antibiotics in dermatology. *Arch. Dermatol.* 1988; 124:1691-1700.

[134] Warner, GT; Plosker, GL. Clindamycin/benzoyl peroxide gel: a review of its use in the management of acne. *Am. J. Clin. Dermatol.* 2002; 3:349-360.

[135] Cunliffe, WJ; Holland, KT; Bojar, R; et al. A randomized, double-blind comparison of a clindamycin phosphate/benzoyl peroxide gel formulation and a matching clindamycin gel with respect to microbiologic activity and clinical efficacy in the topical treatment of acne vulgaris. *Clin. Ther.* 2002; 24:1117-1133.

[136] Tschen, E; Jones, T. A new treatment for acne vulgaris combining benzoyl peroxide with clindamycin. *J. Drugs Dermatol.* 2002; 1:153-157.

[137] Bojar, RA; Eady, EA; Jones, CE; et al. Inhibition of erythromycin-resistant propionibacteria on the skin of acne patients by topical erythromycin with and without zinc. *Br. J. Dermatol.* 1994; 130:329-336.

[138] Gratton, D; Raymond, GP; Guertin-Larochelle, S; et al. Topical clindamycin versus systemic tetracycline in the treatment of acne. Results of a multiclinic trial. *J. Am. Acad. Dermatol.* 1982; 7:50-53.

[139] Leyden, JJ; Shalita, AR; Saatjian, GD; et al. Erythromycin 2% gel in comparison with clindamycin phosphate 1% solution in acne vulgaris. *J. Am. Acad. Dermatol.* 1987; 16:822-827.

[140] Eady, EA; Farmery, MR; Ross, JI; et al. Effects of benzoyl peroxide and erythromycin alone and in combination against antibiotic-sensitive and -resistant skin bacteria from acne patients. *Br. J. Dermatol.* 1994; 131:331-336.

[141] Eady, EA; Bojar, RA; Jones, CE; et al. The effects of acne treatment with a combination of benzoyl peroxide and erythromycin on skin

carriage of erythromycin-resistant propionibacteria. *Br. J. Dermatol.* 1996; 134:107-113.

[142] Borglund, E; Hagermark, O; Nord, CE. Impact of topical clindamycin and systemic tetracycline on the skin and colon microflora in patients with acne vulgaris. *Scand. J. Infect. Dis. Suppl.* 1984; 43:76-81.

[143] Crawford, WW; Crawford, IP; Stoughton, RB; et al. Laboratory induction and clinical occurrence of combined clindamycin and erythromycin resistance in Corynebacterium acnes. *J. Invest. Dermatol.* 1979; 72:187-190.

[144] Eady, EA; Ingham, E; Walters, CE; et al. Modulation of comedonal levels of interleukin-1 in acne patients treated with tetracyclines. *J. Invest. Dermatol.* 1993; 101:86-91.

[145] Dreno, B; Moyse, D; Alirezai, M; et al. Multicenter randomized comparative double-blind controlled clinical trial of the safety and efficacy of zinc gluconate versus minocycline hydrochloride in the treatment of inflammatory acne vulgaris. *Dermatology.* 2001; 203:135-140.

[146] Ochsendorf, F. Systemic antibiotic therapy of acne vulgaris. *J. Deutsch. Dermatol. Ges.* 2006; 4:828-841.

[147] Cleach, LL; Bocquet, H; Roujeau, JC. Reactions and interactions of some commonly used systemic drugs in dermatology. *Dermatol. Clin.* 1998; 16:421-429.

[148] Bacon, JF; Shenfield, GM. Pregnancy attributable to interaction between tetracycline and oral contraceptives. *BMJ.* 1980; 280:293.

[149] Steigbigel, NH; Reed, CW; Finland, M. Susceptibility of common pathogenic bacteria to seven tetracycline antibiotics in vitro. *Am. J. Med. Sci.* 1968; 255:179-195.

[150] Fenske, NA; Millns, JL. Cutaneous pigmentation due to minocycline hydrochloride. *J. Am. Acad. Dermatol.* 1980; 3:308-310.

[151] Caro, I. Discoloration of the teeth related to minocycline therapy for acne. *J. Am. Acad. Dermatol.* 1980; 3:317-318.

[152] Simons, JJ; Morales, A. Minocycline and generalized cutaneous pigmentation. *J. Am. Acad. Dermatol.* 1980; 3:244-247.

[153] Ferner, RE; Moss, C. Minocycline for acne. *BMJ.* 1996; 312:138.

[154] Gottlieb, A. Safety of minocycline for acne. *Lancet.* 1997; 349:374.

[155] Mochizuki, K; Takahashi, T; Kano, M; et al. Pseudotumor cerebri induced by minocycline therapy for acne vulgaris. *Jpn. J. Ophthalmol.* 2002; 46:668-672.

[156] Forti, G; Benincori, C. Doxycycline and the teeth. *Lancet.* 1969; 1:782.

[157] Benjamin, RW; Calikoglu, AS. Hyperthyroidism and lupus-like syndrome in an adolescent treated with minocycline for acne vulgaris. *Pediatr. Dermatol.* 2007; 24:246-249.

[158] Stewart, DM; Torok, HM; Weiss, JS; et al. Dose-ranging efficacy of new once-daily extended-release minocycline for acne vulgaris. *Cutis.* 2006; 78(Suppl 4):11-20.

[159] Garner,SE; Eady, EA; Popescu, C; et al. Minocycline for acne vulgaris: efficacy and safety. *Cochrane Database Syst. Rev.* 2000;(2):CD002086.

[160] Garner, SE; Eady, EA; Popescu, C; et al. Minocycline for acne vulgaris: efficacy and safety. *Cochrane Database Syst. Rev.* 2003;(1):CD002086.

[161] Meyer, FP. Minocycline for acne. Food reduces minocycline's bioavailability. *BMJ.* 1996; 312:1101.

[162] Fernandez-Obregon, AC. Azithromycin for the treatment of acne. *Int. J. Dermatol.* 2000; 39:45-50.

[163] Singhi, MK; Ghiya, BC; Dhabhai, RK. Comparison of oral azithromycin pulse with daily doxycycline in the treatment of acne vulgaris. *Indian J.Dermatol. Venereol. Leprol.* 2003; 69:274-276.

[164] Bottomley, WW; Cunliffe, WJ. Oral trimethoprim as a third-line antibiotic in the management of acne vulgaris. *Dermatology.* 1993; 187:193-196.

[165] Thiboutot, D; Chen, W. Update and future of hormonal therapy in acne. *Dermatology.* 2003; 206:57-67.

[166] Lucky, AW; Koltun, W; Thiboutot, D; et al. A combined oral contraceptive containing 3-mg drospirenone/ 20-microg ethinyl estradiol in the treatment of acne vulgaris: a randomized, double-blind, placebo-controlled study evaluating lesion counts and participant self-assessment. *Cutis.* 2008; 82:143-150.

[167] Thielitz, A; Krautheim, A; Gollnick, H. Update in retinoid therapy of acne. *Dermatol. Ther.* 2006; 19:272-279.

[168] Kligman, AM. The growing importance of topical retinoids in clinical dermatology: a retrospective and prospective analysis. *J. Am. Acad. Dermatol.*1998; 39:S2-S7.

[169] Webster, GF; MD, P. Safety and Efficacy of Tretin-X Compared With Retin-A in Patients With Mild-to-Severe Acne Vulgaris. *SKINmed.* 2006; 5:114-118.

[170] Irby, CE; Yentzer, BA; Feldman, SR. A review of adapalene in the treatment of acne vulgaris. *J. Adoles. Health.* 2008; 43:421-424.

[171] Zaenglein, AL. Topical retinoids in the treatment of acne vulgaris. *Semin.Cutan. Med. Surg.* 2008; 27:177-182.

[172] Jick, SS; Terris, BZ; Jick, H. First trimester topical tretinoin and congenital disorders. *Lancet.* 1993; 341:1181-1182.

[173] Leyden, JJ. Topical treatment of acne vulgaris: retinoids and cutaneous irritation. *J. Am. Acad. Dermatol.* 1998; 38:S1-S4.

[174] Ioannides, D; Rigopoulos, D; Katsambas, A. Topical adapalene gel 0.1% vs. isotretinoin gel 0.05% in the treatment of acne vulgaris: a randomized open-label clinical trial. *Br. J. Dermatol.* 2002; 147:523-527.

[175] Shalita, AR; Chalker, DK; Griffith, RF; et al. Tazarotene gel is safe and effective in the treatment of acne vulgaris: a multicenter, double-blind, vehicle-controlled study. *Cutis.* 1999; 63(6):349-354.

[176] Bershad, S; Kranjac, SG; Parente, JE; et al. Successful treatment of acne vulgaris using a new method: results of a randomized vehicle-controlled trial of short-contact therapy with 0.1% tazarotene gel. *Arch. Dermatol.* 2002; 138:481-489.

[177] Leyden, JJ; Tanghetti, EA; Miller, B; et al. Once-daily tazarotene 0.1 % gel versus once-daily tretinoin 0.1 % microsponge gel for the treatment of facial acne vulgaris: a double-blind randomized trial. *Cutis.* 2002; 69(Suppl 2):12-19.

[178] Pariser, D; Colon, LE; Johnson, LA; et al. Adapalene 0.1% gel compared to tazarotene 0.1% cream in the treatment of acne vulgaris. *J. Drugs Dermatol.* 2008; 7(Suppl 6):S18-S23.

[179] Thiboutot, D; Arsonnaud, S; Soto, P. Efficacy and tolerability of adapalene 0.3% gel compared to tazarotene 0.1% gel in the treatment of acne vulgaris. *J.Drugs Dermatol.* 2008; 7(Suppl 6):S3-S10.

[180] Marazzi, P; Boorman, GC; Donald, AE; et al. Clinical evaluation of Double Strength Isotrexin versus Benzamycin in the topical treatment of mild to moderate acne vulgaris. *J. Dermatolog. Treat.* 2002; 13:111-117.

[181] Draelos, ZD; Tanghetti, EA. Tazarotene Combination Leads to Efficacious Acne Results. Optimizing the use of tazarotene for the treatment of facial acne vulgaris through combination therapy. *Cutis.* 2002; 69(Suppl 2):20-29.

[182] Gold, LS; Colon, LE; Johnson, LA; et al. Is switching retinoids a sound strategy for the treatment of acne vulgaris? *J. Drugs Dermatol.* 2008; 7(Suppl 6):S11-S17.

[183] Cunliffe, WJ; van de Kerkhof, PC; Caputo, R; et al. Roaccutane treatment guidelines: results of an international survey. *Dermatology.* 1997; 194:351-357.

[184] Mallon, E; Newton, JN; Klassen, A; et al. The quality of life in acne: a comparison with general medical conditions using generic questionnaires. *Br. J. Dermatol.* 1999; 140:672-676.

[185] Goulden, V; Clark, SM; McGeown, C; et al. Treatment of acne with intermittent isotretinoin. *Br. J. Dermatol.* 1997; 137:106-108.

[186] Akman, A; Durusoy, C; Senturk, M; et al. Treatment of acne with intermittent and conventional isotretinoin: a randomized, controlled multicenter study. *Arch. Dermatolog. Res.* 2007; 299:467-473.

[187] Holmes, S; Bankowska, U; Mackie, RM. The prescription of isotretinoin to women: is every precaution taken? *Br. J. Dermatol.* 1998; 138:450-455.

[188] Kawada, A; Aragane, Y; Kameyama, H; et al. Acne phototherapy with a high-intensity, enhanced, narrow-band, blue light source: an open study and in vitro investigation. *J. Dermatolog. Sci.* 2002; 30:129-135.

[189] Margolis, DJ; Attie, M; Leyden, JJ. Effects of isotretinoin on bone mineralization during routine therapy with isotretinoin for acne vulgaris. *Arch.Dermatol.*1996; 132:769-774.

[190] Goulden, V; Layton, AM; Cunliffe, WJ. Current indications for isotretinoin as a treatment for acne vulgaris. *Dermatology.* 1995; 190:284-287.

[191] Berard, A; Azoulay, L; Koren, G; et al. Isotretinoin, pregnancies, abortions and birth defects: a population-based perspective. *Br. J. Clin. Pharmacol.* 2007; 63:196-205.

[192] Ng, CH; Tam, MM; Celi, E; et al. Prospective study of depressive symptoms and quality of life in acne vulgaris patients treated with isotretinoin compared to antibiotic and topical therapy. *Aust. J. Dermatol.* 2002; 43:262-268.

[193] Charakida, A; Seaton, ED; Charakida, M; et al. Phototherapy in the treatment of acne vulgaris: what is its role? *Am. J. Clin. Dermatol.* 2004; 5:211-216.

[194] Munavalli, GS; Weiss, RA. Evidence for laser- and light-based treatment of acne vulgaris. *Semin. Cutan. Med. Surg.* 2008; 27:207-211.

[195] Dreno, B. Acne: physical treatment. *Clin. Dermatol.* 2004; 22:429-433.

[196] Papageorgiou, P; Katsambas, A; Chu, A. Phototherapy with blue (415 nm) and red (660 nm) light in the treatment of acne vulgaris. *Br. J. Dermatol.* 2000; 142:973-978.

[197] Na, JI; Suh, DH. Red light phototherapy alone is effective for acne vulgaris: randomized, single-blinded clinical trial. *Dermatol. Surg.* 2007; 33:1228-1233.

[198] Genina, EA; Bashkatov, AN; Simonenko, GV; et al. Low-intensity indocyanine-green laser phototherapy of acne vulgaris: pilot study. *J. Biomed. Optics* 2004; 9:828-834.

[199] Goldberg, DJ; Russell, BA. Combination blue (415 nm) and red (633 nm) LED phototherapy in the treatment of mild to severe acne vulgaris. *J. Cos.Laser Ther.* 2006; 8:71-75.

[200] Lee, SY; You, CE; Park, MY. Blue and red light combination LED phototherapy for acne vulgaris in patients with skin phototype IV. *Lasers Surg. Med.* 2007; 39:180-188.

[201] Zane, C; Capezzera, R; Pedretti, A; et al. Non-invasive diagnostic evaluation of phototherapeutic effects of red light phototherapy of acne vulgaris. *Photodermatol. Photoimmunol. Photomed.* 2008; 24:244-248.

[202] Ammad, S; Gonzales, M; Edwards, C; et al. An assessment of the efficacy of blue light phototherapy in the treatment of acne vulgaris. *J. Cos. Dermatol.* 2008; 7:180-188.

[203] Wiegell, SR; Wulf, HC. Photodynamic therapy of acne vulgaris using methyl aminolaevulinate: a blinded, randomized, controlled trial. *Br. J. Dermatol.* 2006; 154:969-976.

[204] Nouri, K; Villafradez-Diaz, LM. Light/laser therapy in the treatment of acne vulgaris. *J. Cos. Dermatol.* 2005; 4:318-320.

[205] Orringer, JS; Kang, S; Hamilton, T; et al. Treatment of acne vulgaris with a pulsed dye laser: a randomized controlled trial. *JAMA.* 2004; 291:2834-2839.

[206] Baugh, WP; Kucaba, WD. Nonablative phototherapy for acne vulgaris using the KTP 532 nm laser. *Dermatol. Surg.* 2005; 31:1290-1296.

[207] Lihong, S. He-Ne laser auricular irradiation plus body acupuncture for treatment of acne vulgaris in 36 cases. *J. Trad. Chin. Med.* 2006; 26:193-194.

[208] Sami, NA; Attia, AT; Badawi, AM. Phototherapy in the treatment of acne vulgaris. *J. Drugs Dermatol.* 2008; 7:627-632.

[209] Levine, RM; Rasmussen, JE. Intralesional corticosteroids in the treatment of nodulocystic acne. *Arch. Dermatol.* 1983; 119:480-481.

[210] Shalita, AR; Smith, JG; Parish, LC; et al. Topical nicotinamide compared with clindamycin gel in the treatment of inflammatory acne vulgaris. *Int. J. Dermatol.* 1995; 34:434-437.

[211] Sardesai, VR; Kambli, VM. Comparison of efficacy of topical clindamycin and nicotinamide combination with plain clindamycin for the treatment of acne vulgaris and acne resistant to topical antibiotics. *Indian J. Dermatol.Venereol. Leprol.* 2003; 69:138-139.

[212] Dos, SK; Barbhuiya, JN; Jana, S; et al. Comparative evaluation of clindamycin phosphate 1% and clindamycin phosphate 1% with nicotinamide gel 4% in the treatment of acne vulgaris. *Indian J. Dermatol. Venereol. Leprol.* 2003; 69:8-9.

[213] Dreno, B; Amblard, P; Agache, P; et al. Low doses of zinc gluconate for inflammatory acne. *Acta Derm. Venereol.* 1989; 69:541-543.

[214] Klock, J; Ikeno, H; Ohmori, K; et al. Sodium ascorbyl phosphate shows in vitro and in vivo efficacy in the prevention and treatment of acne vulgaris. *Int. J. Cos. Sci.* 2005; 27:171-176.

[215] Kim, J. Acne vaccines: therapeutic option for the treatment of acne vulgaris? *J. Invest. Dermatol.* 2008; 128:2353-2354.

[216] Zouboulis, CC; Piquero-Martin, J. Update and future of systemic acne treatment. Dermatology. 2003; 206:37-53.

[217] Layton, AM; Henderson, CA; Cunliffe, WJ. A clinical evaluation of acne scarring and its incidence. *Clin. Exp. Dermatol.* 1994; 19:303-308.

[218] Lucky, AW; Biro, FM; Simbartl, LA; et al. Predictors of severity of acne vulgaris in young adolescent girls: results of a five-year longitudinal study. *J. Pediatr.* 1997; 130:30-39.

[219] Motley, RJ; Finlay, AY. Practical use of a disability index in the routine management of acne. *Clin. Exp. Dermatol.* 1992; 17:1-3.

[220] Keri, JE. Acne: improving skin and self-esteem. *Pediatr. Ann.* 2006; 35:174-179.

[221] Leaute-Labreze, C; Gautier, C; Labbe, L; et al. Infantile acne and isotretinoin. *Ann. Dermatol. Venereol.* 1998; 125:132-134.

[222] Sarazin, F; Dompmartin, A; Nivot, S; et al. Treatment of an infantile acne with oral isotretinoin. *Eur. J. Dermatol.* 2004; 14:71-72.

[223] Barnes, CJ; Eichenfield, LF; Lee, J; et al. A practical approach for the use of oral isotretinoin for infantile acne. *Pediatr. Dermatol.* 2005; 22:166-169.

INDEX

antibiotic, vii, 34, 36, 38, 39, 55, 56, 57, 61, 72, 73, 74, 76
antibiotic resistance, 36, 38, 39, 61
antibiotics, vii, 34, 35, 36, 37, 38, 47, 55, 59, 61, 72, 73, 77
anticoagulants, 38
anticonvulsants, 38
anti-inflammatory agents, 57
antisense, 57
anxiety, vii, 31, 59, 63
anxiety disorder, 32
arthralgia, 46, 54
arthritis, 31, 60
assessment, 15, 16, 25, 27, 39, 40, 48, 68, 77
assignment, 52
asthma, 60
athletes, 29
atopic dermatitis, 71
atrophy, 54
Australia, 3
averaging, 45
avoidance, 17, 33

B

babies, 46
back, vii, 1, 5, 9, 19, 20, 51, 60, 61
back pain, 60
bacteria, 8, 10, 48, 72, 73
bacterial, 35, 36, 39, 52, 57, 61
bacterial strains, 61
bacteriophage, 57, 65
behavior, 70
beliefs, 19
beneficial effect, 4
benefits, 46
benign, 38, 45
benzoyl peroxide, vii, 34, 35, 36, 37, 40, 43, 44, 48, 55, 59, 61, 72
binding, 16, 17, 38, 41
binding globulin, 16, 17
bioavailability, 74
biological activity, 17
biological responses, 15

biopsies, 45
birth, 11, 46, 76
blood, 16, 18, 69
blood glucose, 16
bloodstream, 18
body mass, 14
body mass index, 14
bovine, 14, 54
boys, 3, 5, 15, 20, 59, 66
brassieres, 9
breakfast, 14
bulbs, 47
burning, 41, 42, 43, 44, 52
butterfly, 23

C

calcium, 38
candidiasis, 23
carbohydrate, 16, 17
carbohydrates, 15, 16, 17
carcinogenic, 41, 52
carrier, 55
Caucasians, 5
causal inference, 32
causal relationship, 47
causation, 18
cell, 7, 11, 40, 65
cell growth, 11
cheese, 14, 18
cheilitis, 46
chemotaxis, 37
chest, 1, 5, 19, 20
childbearing, 46
childhood, 24
children, 2, 5, 20, 37, 38, 59, 64, 71
China, 4
chloride, 61
chlorine, 2
chocolate, 16, 33, 66
cigarettes, 13
CINAHL, 18
cis, 41, 45, 69, 70
citizens, 13
classification, 19

H

I

T